MW00532789

THE BEDTIME JOURNAL

Two Minutes Each Night for Restful Sleep

LEAHANNE THOMAS

STERLING
New York

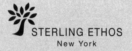

STERLING ETHOS
New York

STERLING ETHOS and the distinctive Sterling Ethos logo are registered
trademarks of Sterling Publishing Co., Inc.

Text © 2022 Leahanne Thomas

ISBN 978-1-4549-4618-2

Distributed in Canada by Sterling Publishing Co., Inc.
c/o Canadian Manda Group, 664 Annette Street
Toronto, Ontario, Canada M6S 2C8
Distributed in the United Kingdom by GMC Distribution Services
Castle Place, 166 High Street, Lewes, East Sussex, England BN7 1XU
Distributed in Australia by NewSouth Books
University of New South Wales, Sydney, NSW 2052, Australia

For information about custom editions, special sales, and premium purchases,
please contact specialsales@sterlingpublishing.com.

Printed in Malaysia

2 4 6 8 10 9 7 5 3 1

www.sterlingpublishing.com

Design by Jordan Wannemacher

Cover and interior illustrations by Maggie Enterrios
Cover design by Melissa Farris

FOR A GOOD NIGHT'S SLEEP

Have you ever tried to go to sleep and found you couldn't because your mind was racing? Thoughts about what you wish you'd done differently that day or thoughts about what's ahead of you tomorrow run wild, keeping you awake, restless, and stressed.

The *Bedtime Journal* was created to help you get a good night's sleep. Pure and simple. Something magical happens when thoughts move from your head to paper—they stop being monsters consuming you and they turn into manageable concepts.

How does the book work? It sits on your nightstand, and you write for five minutes every night before you turn out the lights. It's structured—you answer the same four questions every day—but at the same time, it's flexible. It is meant to be quick and painless. No one wants to do a lot of work before they go to sleep; that defeats the purpose.

Each day has four boxes that are "quick hits." The first two are to take stock of your day and then put it to rest. The first box is for acknowledging at least one success or one happiness for the day. It can be large or small, one or many. But everyone has at least one success or moment of joy every day. Acknowledging our successes and joys reminds us that every day is a gift and to be grateful for what we have accomplished this day. Our life should not be taken for granted or overlooked.

The second box is for the mistakes, missteps, failures, or redos. To err is human and yet we humans struggle with our errors. We either deny them or make them larger than they truly are. They can be large or small—eating too many cookies, blowing a deal, not studying for a test, being impatient with another person. Write it down, acknowledge it and "put it to bed." Some days are better than others; some days you may have four mess-ups and other days none. Life is messy, but not recognizing our missteps keeps us up at night.

Then on to tomorrow. What do you hope to accomplish and why? Tomorrow is not guaranteed to any of us, but if you're lucky enough to be granted another day, what one thing would you like to accomplish—big or small? Research shows that we're more likely to complete something if we know why we're doing it. So, there's a checkbox for you to acknowledge your "why."

The weekend is an opportunity to take stock of the week. Often, we manage our lives like to-do lists, and we don't stop to acknowledge where we are and where you're going. The weekend is a good time to check in on how our week went. You have reflection space to note your big success of the week—what stood out to you this week. What was your best experience? It could be different from a success. Weekends are when we relax and recharge, so what treat did you give yourself this weekend? It could be as simple as a walk in the woods or a good movie. And, lastly, what inspiration or realization did you have this week? Perhaps you closed a chapter on an issue or opened a new door.

Quarterly, there are reflection pages to look back over the previous few months. What, if anything, has changed for you since you have been more intentional in your life? Maybe you see things differently or have a new focus. What themes have been recurring?

Maybe you've had the same recurring misstep. Is it time to change anything? Is there something you could do differently to get different results?

And that's it. If you commit to five minutes every night just before you turn out the lights, you will sleep better, feel better, and feel a sense of growth and progress.

I hope you like it; I made it for you.

—LEAHANNE

"If you don't design your own life plan, chances are you'll fall into someone else's plan. And guess what they have planned for you? Not much."
—JIM ROHN

DATE: __/__/__

One success I had today:

One redo I want:

One goal for tomorrow:

Why:

- ☐ Make others happy
- ☐ Show love and support
- ☐ Challenge myself
- ☐ Feel good/have fun
- ☐ Complete overdue task
- ☐ Resolve something
- ☐ Make progress
- ☐ Relax

TUESDAY

DATE: 1/2/23

"Humor is the great thing, the saving thing. The minute it crops up, all our hardnesses yield." —**MARK TWAIN**

One happiness today:

Defenitly the Sunrise up at Snow Bowl Hut

One screwup:

Not realizing I had Hw in CHEM until 10min before it was due. ☺ Had to really rush it.

One intention for tomorrow:

Crush all my classes, & start this quarter off right

Why:

- [ ] Make others happy
- [ ] Show love and support
- [x] Challenge myself
- [x] Feel good/have fun
- [ ] Complete overdue task
- [ ] Resolve something
- [x] Make progress
- [ ] Relax

"Indeed is not everything impossible until it is done?"—**DANIEL WILSON**

DATE: __/__/__

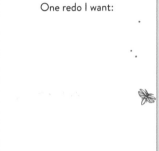

One success I had today:

One redo I want:

One goal for tomorrow:

Why:

- ☐ Make others happy
- ☐ Show love and support
- ☐ Challenge myself
- ☐ Feel good/have fun
- ☐ Complete overdue task
- ☐ Resolve something
- ☐ Make progress
- ☐ Relax

*"Once you accept the universe as matter expanding
into nothing that is something, wearing stripes
with plaid comes easy."*
—ATTRIBUTED TO ALBERT EINSTEIN

THURSDAY

DATE: __/__/__

One happiness today:

Realizing its my Friday & I just make it through my first week! Only 11 more to go! Also I started reading the screenplay for Blade Runner 2049 Its Fire!!!!

One screwup:

I didn't watch the video lectures of Ch 2 & 3 before the quiz on it in Bio. I only studied the slides "...

One intention for tomorrow:

To start training for the Tacoma Marathon in April

Why:

- ☐ Make others happy
- ☐ Show love and support
- ☒ Challenge myself
- ☒ Feel good/have fun
- ☒ Complete overdue task
- ☒ Resolve something
- ☒ Make progress
- ☐ Relax

FRIDAY

DATE: 61/05 2024

"Perseverance is not a long race; it is many short races one after the other."—**WALTER ELLIOTT**

One success I had today:

Finishing my chem Hw

One redo I want:

I wish I would've ran...

One goal for tomorrow:

Attend the protest for Palestine

Why

- ☐ Make others happy
- ☒ Show love and support
- ☐ Challenge myself
- ☐ Feel good/have fun
- ☐ Complete overdue task
- ☒ Resolve something
- ☒ Make progress
- ☐ Relax

"If a book about failures doesn't sell, is it a success?" —JERRY SEINFELD

Success of the week:

The christmas/going away party was a huge hit & everyone had a great time! :)

Best experience of the week:

The ferry ride w/ mateo & jake on Tues was so, so, so, beautiful. It went from Bremerton to Seattle. 10/10 jmust do again !!!

One treat planned for the weekend:

Me & Jake are going snowshoing into the backcountry to Burley Mtn Lookout & are gonna stay the night for the New Year!

One inspiration/realization:

This week I've truly lived & have been trying my hardest to embody "Carpe Diem" "Seize the Day"

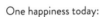

"Problems are not stop signs, they are guidelines."
—ROBERT H. SCHULLER

One happiness today:

Seeing Poor Things, a second time & loving it again!!

One screwup:

Not watching Ch 6 lecture before BIO, I was so so so Lost 😤😤

One intention for tomorrow:

Pickup couch from lili's place & move stuff to storage unit

Why:

☐ Make others happy
☐ Show love & support
☐ Challenge myself
☐ Feel good/have fun
☐ Complete overdue task
☐ Resolve something
☑ Make progress
☐ Relax

DATE: 1/9/24

*"Make it thy business to know thyself, which is the
most difficult lesson in the world."*
—MIGUEL DE CERVANTES

One success I had today:

Starting to
move finally

One redo I want:

I shouldve done
more HW & studie
more

One goal for tomorrow:

Workout!!!

Why:

☐ Make others happy
☐ Show love & support
☒ Challenge myself
☐ Feel good/have fun
☒ Complete overdue task
☐ Resolve something
☒ Make progress
☐ Relax

WEDNESDAY

"Ever tried. Ever failed. No matter. Try Again. Fail again. Fail Better." **—SAMUEL BECKETT**

One happiness today:

One screwup:

One intention for tomorrow:

Why:

- ☐ Make others happy
- ☐ Show love & support
- ☐ Challenge myself
- ☐ Feel good/have fun
- ☐ Complete overdue task
- ☐ Resolve something
- ☐ Make progress
- ☐ Relax

THURSDAY

DATE: __/__/__

"It ain't over till it's over." —**YOGI BERRA**

One success I had today:

One redo I want:

One goal for tomorrow:

Why:

☐ Make others happy
☐ Show love & support
☐ Challenge myself
☐ Feel good/have fun
☐ Complete overdue task
☐ Resolve something
☐ Make progress
☐ Relax

FRIDAY

DATE: __/__/__

"By leadership, we mean the art of getting someone else to do something you want done because he wants to do it." —**DWIGHT D. EISENHOWER**

One happiness today:

One screwup:

One intention for tomorrow:

Why:

- ☐ Make others happy
- ☐ Show love & support
- ☐ Challenge myself
- ☐ Feel good/have fun
- ☐ Complete overdue task
- ☐ Resolve something
- ☐ Make progress
- ☐ Relax

"Never miss a good chance to shut up."
—WILL ROGERS

Success of the week:

Best experience of the week:

One treat planned for the weekend:

One inspiration/realization:

MONDAY

DATE: __/__/__

"When you reach the end of your rope, tie a knot in it and hang on." —**ANONYMOUS**

One success I had today:

One redo I want:

One goal for tomorrow:

Why:

- ☐ Make others happy
- ☐ Show love & support
- ☐ Challenge myself
- ☐ Feel good/have fun
- ☐ Complete overdue task
- ☐ Resolve something
- ☐ Make progress
- ☐ Relax

TUESDAY

DATE: __/__/__

"Puns are the highest form of literature."
—ALFRED HITCHCOCK

One happiness today:

One screwup:

One intention for tomorrow:

Why:

- [ ] Make others happy
- [ ] Show love & support
- [ ] Challenge myself
- [ ] Feel good/have fun
- [ ] Complete overdue task
- [ ] Resolve something
- [ ] Make progress
- [ ] Relax

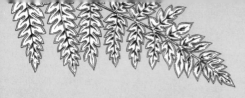

DATE: __/__/__

"I avoid looking forward or backward, and try to keep looking upward." —**CHARLOTTE BRONTË**

One success I had today:

One redo I want:

One goal for tomorrow:

Why:
- ☐ Make others happy
- ☐ Show love & support
- ☐ Challenge myself
- ☐ Feel good/have fun
- ☐ Complete overdue task
- ☐ Resolve something
- ☐ Make progress
- ☐ Relax

THURSDAY

"I live in my own little world. But it's OK, they know me here." —**JOEL HODGSON**

One happiness today:

One screwup:

One intention for tomorrow:

Why:
- ☐ Make others happy
- ☐ Show love & support
- ☐ Challenge myself
- ☐ Feel good/have fun
- ☐ Complete overdue task
- ☐ Resolve something
- ☐ Make progress
- ☐ Relax

"Only I can change my life. No one can do it for me."—**CAROL BURNETT**

DATE: __/__/__

One success I had today:

One redo I want:

One goal for tomorrow:

Why:

☐ Make others happy
☐ Show love & support
☐ Challenge myself
☐ Feel good/have fun
☐ Complete overdue task
☐ Resolve something
☐ Make progress
☐ Relax

"To rank the effort above the prize may be called love." —**CONFUCIUS**

DATE: __/__/__

Success of the week:

Best experience of the week:

One treat planned for the weekend:

One inspiration/realization:

"I can, therefore I am." —SIMONE WEIL

One happiness today:

One screwup:

One intention for tomorrow:

Why:

- ☐ Make others happy
- ☐ Show love & support
- ☐ Challenge myself
- ☐ Feel good/have fun
- ☐ Complete overdue task
- ☐ Resolve something
- ☐ Make progress
- ☐ Relax

"Happiness is doing it rotten your way."
—ISAAC ASIMOV

DATE: __/__/__

One success I had today:

One redo I want:

One goal for tomorrow:

Why:

☐ Make others happy
☐ Show love & support
☐ Challenge myself
☐ Feel good/have fun
☐ Complete overdue task
☐ Resolve something
☐ Make progress
☐ Relax

DATE: __/__/__

"Expect problems and eat them for breakfast."
—ALFRED A. MONTAPERT

One happiness today:

One screwup:

One intention for tomorrow:

Why:

☐ Make others happy
☐ Show love & support
☐ Challenge myself
☐ Feel good/have fun
☐ Complete overdue task
☐ Resolve something
☐ Make progress
☐ Relax

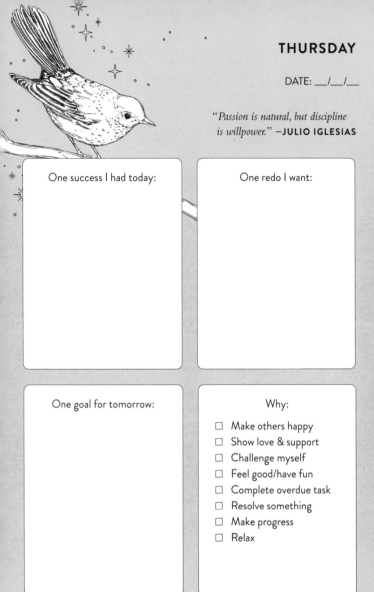

THURSDAY

DATE: __/__/__

"Passion is natural, but discipline is willpower." —**JULIO IGLESIAS**

One success I had today:

One redo I want:

One goal for tomorrow:

Why:

- ☐ Make others happy
- ☐ Show love & support
- ☐ Challenge myself
- ☐ Feel good/have fun
- ☐ Complete overdue task
- ☐ Resolve something
- ☐ Make progress
- ☐ Relax

FRIDAY

DATE: __/__/__

"Leap, and the net will appear."
—JOHN BURROUGHS

One happiness today:

One screwup:

One intention for tomorrow:

Why:

- ☐ Make others happy
- ☐ Show love & support
- ☐ Challenge myself
- ☐ Feel good/have fun
- ☐ Complete overdue task
- ☐ Resolve something
- ☐ Make progress
- ☐ Relax

"Never trust people who smile constantly. They're either selling something or not very bright."
—LAURELL K. HAMILTON

DATE: __/__/__

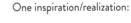

Success of the week:

Best experience of the week:

One treat planned for the weekend:

One inspiration/realization:

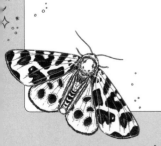

"If you want to succeed you should strike out new paths, rather than travel the worn paths of accepted success." —**JOHN D. ROCKEFELLER**

DATE: __/__/__

One success I had today:

One redo I want:

One goal for tomorrow:

Why:

- ☐ Make others happy
- ☐ Show love & support
- ☐ Challenge myself
- ☐ Feel good/have fun
- ☐ Complete overdue task
- ☐ Resolve something
- ☐ Make progress
- ☐ Relax

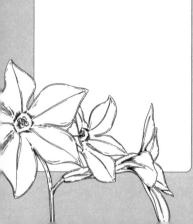

"If at first you don't succeed, then skydiving definitely isn't for you." —**STEVEN WRIGHT**

DATE: __/__/__

One happiness today:

One screwup:

One intention for tomorrow:

Why:

- ☐ Make others happy
- ☐ Show love & support
- ☐ Challenge myself
- ☐ Feel good/have fun
- ☐ Complete overdue task
- ☐ Resolve something
- ☐ Make progress
- ☐ Relax

"Set your goals high, and don't stop until you get there." **—BO JACKSON**

DATE: __/__/__

One success I had today:

One redo I want:

One goal for tomorrow:

Why:

- ☐ Make others happy
- ☐ Show love & support
- ☐ Challenge myself
- ☐ Feel good/have fun
- ☐ Complete overdue task
- ☐ Resolve something
- ☐ Make progress
- ☐ Relax

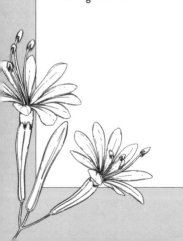

"Man needs difficulties; they are necessary for health."
—CARL JUNG

One happiness today:

One screwup:

One intention for tomorrow:

Why:

- ☐ Make others happy
- ☐ Show love & support
- ☐ Challenge myself
- ☐ Feel good/have fun
- ☐ Complete overdue task
- ☐ Resolve something
- ☐ Make progress
- ☐ Relax

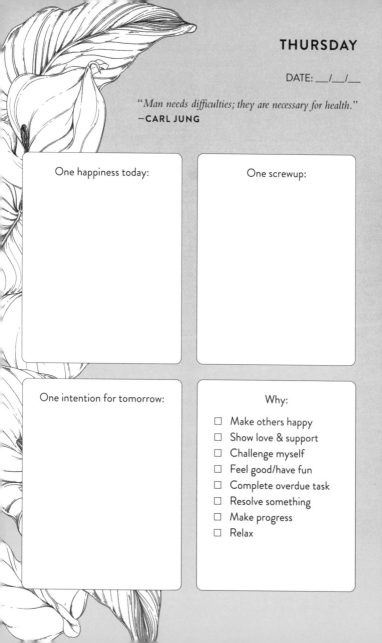

"Life is 10 percent what happens to you and 90 percent how you react to it."
—CHARLES R. SWINDOLL

DATE: __/__/__

One success I had today:

One redo I want:

One goal for tomorrow:

Why:

- [ ] Make others happy
- [ ] Show love & support
- [ ] Challenge myself
- [ ] Feel good/have fun
- [ ] Complete overdue task
- [ ] Resolve something
- [ ] Make progress
- [ ] Relax

DATE: __/__/__

"I've always wanted to go to Switzerland to see what the army does with those wee red knives." **—BILLY CONNOLLY**

Success of the week:

Best experience of the week:

One treat planned for the weekend:

One inspiration/realization:

*"Good, better, best. Never let it rest. 'Til our good
is better and our better is best."*
—ANONYMOUS

DATE: __/__/__

One happiness today:

One screwup:

One intention for tomorrow:

Why:

- ☐ Make others happy
- ☐ Show love & support
- ☐ Challenge myself
- ☐ Feel good/have fun
- ☐ Complete overdue task
- ☐ Resolve something
- ☐ Make progress
- ☐ Relax

"The suspense is terrible. I hope it will last."
—OSCAR WILDE

DATE: __/__/__

One success I had today:

One redo I want:

One goal for tomorrow:

Why:

- ☐ Make others happy
- ☐ Show love & support
- ☐ Challenge myself
- ☐ Feel good/have fun
- ☐ Complete overdue task
- ☐ Resolve something
- ☐ Make progress
- ☐ Relax

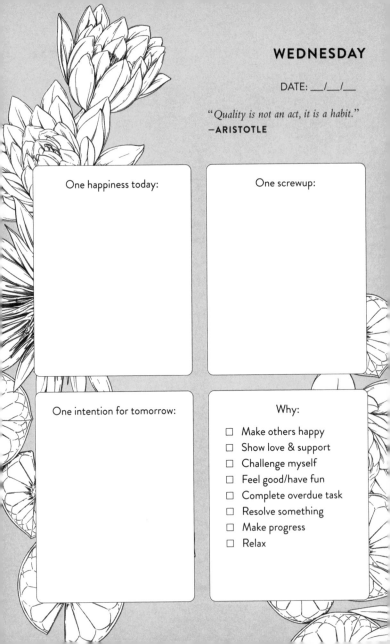

WEDNESDAY

DATE: __/__/__

"Quality is not an act, it is a habit."
—ARISTOTLE

One happiness today:

One screwup:

One intention for tomorrow:

Why:

- ☐ Make others happy
- ☐ Show love & support
- ☐ Challenge myself
- ☐ Feel good/have fun
- ☐ Complete overdue task
- ☐ Resolve something
- ☐ Make progress
- ☐ Relax

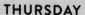

"Knowledge is like underwear. It is useful to have, but not necessary to show it off."
—BILL MURRAY

One success I had today:

One redo I want:

One goal for tomorrow:

Why:

- ☐ Make others happy
- ☐ Show love & support
- ☐ Challenge myself
- ☐ Feel good/have fun
- ☐ Complete overdue task
- ☐ Resolve something
- ☐ Make progress
- ☐ Relax

"With the new day comes new strength and new thoughts." —ELEANOR ROOSEVELT

DATE: ___/___/___

One happiness today:

One screwup:

One intention for tomorrow:

Why:

- ☐ Make others happy
- ☐ Show love & support
- ☐ Challenge myself
- ☐ Feel good/have fun
- ☐ Complete overdue task
- ☐ Resolve something
- ☐ Make progress
- ☐ Relax

"Being entirely honest with oneself is a good exercise."—**SIGMUND FREUD**

DATE: __/__/__

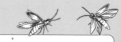

Success of the week:

Best experience of the week:

One treat planned for the weekend:

One inspiration/realization:

DATE: __/__/__

"When something is important enough, you do it even if the odds are not in your favor."
—ELON MUSK

One success I had today:

One redo I want:

One goal for tomorrow:

Why:

- ☐ Make others happy
- ☐ Show love & support
- ☐ Challenge myself
- ☐ Feel good/have fun
- ☐ Complete overdue task
- ☐ Resolve something
- ☐ Make progress
- ☐ Relax

"Happiness is not a goal, it is a by-product."
—ELEANOR ROOSEVELT

One happiness today:

One screwup:

One intention for tomorrow:

Why:

- ☐ Make others happy
- ☐ Show love & support
- ☐ Challenge myself
- ☐ Feel good/have fun
- ☐ Complete overdue task
- ☐ Resolve something
- ☐ Make progress
- ☐ Relax

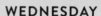

WEDNESDAY

DATE: __/__/__

"Every exit is an entry somewhere else."
—TOM STOPPARD

One success I had today:

One redo I want:

One goal for tomorrow:

Why:

☐ Make others happy
☐ Show love & support
☐ Challenge myself
☐ Feel good/have fun
☐ Complete overdue task
☐ Resolve something
☐ Make progress
☐ Relax

"I hold the maxim no less applicable to public than to private affairs, that honesty is always the best policy." **—GEORGE WASHINGTON**

DATE: __/__/__

One happiness today:

One screwup:

One intention for tomorrow:

Why:

- ☐ Make others happy
- ☐ Show love & support
- ☐ Challenge myself
- ☐ Feel good/have fun
- ☐ Complete overdue task
- ☐ Resolve something
- ☐ Make progress
- ☐ Relax

DATE: __/__/__

"If you fell down yesterday, stand up today."
—H. G. WELLS

One success I had today:

One redo I want:

One goal for tomorrow:

Why:

- ☐ Make others happy
- ☐ Show love & support
- ☐ Challenge myself
- ☐ Feel good/have fun
- ☐ Complete overdue task
- ☐ Resolve something
- ☐ Make progress
- ☐ Relax

DATE: __/__/__

"The four most beautiful words in our common language: I told you so." **—GORE VIDAL**

Success of the week:

Best experience of the week:

One treat planned for the weekend:

One inspiration/realization:

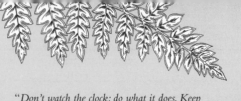

"Don't watch the clock; do what it does. Keep going." —**SAM LEVENSON**

One happiness today:

One screwup:

One intention for tomorrow:

Why:

- ☐ Make others happy
- ☐ Show love & support
- ☐ Challenge myself
- ☐ Feel good/have fun
- ☐ Complete overdue task
- ☐ Resolve something
- ☐ Make progress
- ☐ Relax

"I don't believe you have to be better than everybody else. I believe you have to be better than you ever thought you could be."
—KEN VENTURI

One success I had today:

One redo I want:

One goal for tomorrow:

Why:

- ☐ Make others happy
- ☐ Show love & support
- ☐ Challenge myself
- ☐ Feel good/have fun
- ☐ Complete overdue task
- ☐ Resolve something
- ☐ Make progress
- ☐ Relax

"The only way to keep your health is to eat what you don't want, drink what you don't like, and do what you'd rather not." —**MARK TWAIN**

One happiness today:

One screwup:

One intention for tomorrow:

Why:

☐ Make others happy
☐ Show love & support
☐ Challenge myself
☐ Feel good/have fun
☐ Complete overdue task
☐ Resolve something
☐ Make progress
☐ Relax

"Be kind whenever possible. It is always possible."
—TENZIN GYATSO, THE 14TH DALAI LAMA

THURSDAY

DATE: __/__/__

One success I had today:

One redo I want:

One goal for tomorrow:

Why:

- ☐ Make others happy
- ☐ Show love & support
- ☐ Challenge myself
- ☐ Feel good/have fun
- ☐ Complete overdue task
- ☐ Resolve something
- ☐ Make progress
- ☐ Relax

DATE: __/__/__

"If you can dream it, you can do it."
—WALT DISNEY

One happiness today:

One screwup:

One intention for tomorrow:

Why:

- ☐ Make others happy
- ☐ Show love & support
- ☐ Challenge myself
- ☐ Feel good/have fun
- ☐ Complete overdue task
- ☐ Resolve something
- ☐ Make progress
- ☐ Relax

"Nothing is at last sacred but the integrity of your own mind." —**RALPH WALDO EMERSON**

WEEKEND

DATE: __/__/__

Success of the week:

Best experience of the week:

One treat planned for the weekend:

One inspiration/realization:

"The key is not the will to win . . . everybody has that. It is the will to prepare to win that is important." —**BOBBY KNIGHT**

One happiness today:

One screwup:

One intention for tomorrow:

Why:

- ☐ Make others happy
- ☐ Show love & support
- ☐ Challenge myself
- ☐ Feel good/have fun
- ☐ Complete overdue task
- ☐ Resolve something
- ☐ Make progress
- ☐ Relax

TUESDAY

DATE: __/__/__

"Never go to bed mad. Stay up and fight."
—PHYLLIS DILLER

One success I had today:

One redo I want:

One goal for tomorrow:

Why:

- ☐ Make others happy
- ☐ Show love & support
- ☐ Challenge myself
- ☐ Feel good/have fun
- ☐ Complete overdue task
- ☐ Resolve something
- ☐ Make progress
- ☐ Relax

WEDNESDAY

DATE: __/__/__

*"Failure will never overtake me if my
determination to succeed is strong enough."*
—OG MANDINO

One happiness today:

One screwup:

One intention for tomorrow:

Why:
- ☐ Make others happy
- ☐ Show love & support
- ☐ Challenge myself
- ☐ Feel good/have fun
- ☐ Complete overdue task
- ☐ Resolve something
- ☐ Make progress
- ☐ Relax

DATE: __/__/__

"Know your own happiness. You want nothing but patience—or give it a more fascinating name, call it hope." **—JANE AUSTEN**

One success I had today:

One redo I want:

One goal for tomorrow:

Why:

- ☐ Make others happy
- ☐ Show love & support
- ☐ Challenge myself
- ☐ Feel good/have fun
- ☐ Complete overdue task
- ☐ Resolve something
- ☐ Make progress
- ☐ Relax

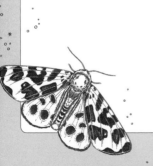

"Start where you are. Use what you have. Do what you can." —**ARTHUR ASHE**

DATE: __/__/__

One happiness today:

One screwup:

One intention for tomorrow:

Why:

- ☐ Make others happy
- ☐ Show love & support
- ☐ Challenge myself
- ☐ Feel good/have fun
- ☐ Complete overdue task
- ☐ Resolve something
- ☐ Make progress
- ☐ Relax

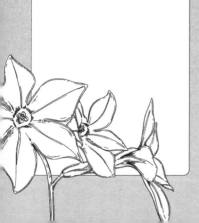

"My life feels like a test I didn't study for."
—ANONYMOUS

DATE: ___/___/___

Success of the week:

Best experience of the week:

One treat planned for the weekend:

One inspiration/realization:

"Even if you fall on your face, you're still moving forward." —**ATTRIBUTED TO VICTOR KIAM**

One success I had today:

One redo I want:

One goal for tomorrow:

Why:

- ☐ Make others happy
- ☐ Show love & support
- ☐ Challenge myself
- ☐ Feel good/have fun
- ☐ Complete overdue task
- ☐ Resolve something
- ☐ Make progress
- ☐ Relax

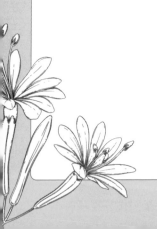

DATE: __/__/__

"Things do not happen. Things are made to happen." —**JOHN F. KENNEDY**

One happiness today:

One screwup:

One intention for tomorrow:

Why:

- ☐ Make others happy
- ☐ Show love & support
- ☐ Challenge myself
- ☐ Feel good/have fun
- ☐ Complete overdue task
- ☐ Resolve something
- ☐ Make progress
- ☐ Relax

> *"The first step toward success is taken when you refuse to be a captive of the environment in which you first find yourself."* **—MARK CAINE**

One success I had today:

One redo I want:

One goal for tomorrow:

Why:

☐ Make others happy
☐ Show love & support
☐ Challenge myself
☐ Feel good/have fun
☐ Complete overdue task
☐ Resolve something
☐ Make progress
☐ Relax

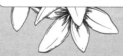

THURSDAY

DATE: __/__/__

"There's a great power in words, if you don't hitch too many of them together."
—JOSH BILLINGS

One happiness today:

One screwup:

One intention for tomorrow:

Why:

- ☐ Make others happy
- ☐ Show love & support
- ☐ Challenge myself
- ☐ Feel good/have fun
- ☐ Complete overdue task
- ☐ Resolve something
- ☐ Make progress
- ☐ Relax

*"Knowing is not enough; we must apply.
Willing is not enough; we must do."*
—JOHANN WOLFGANG VON GOETHE

DATE: ___/___/___

One success I had today:

One redo I want:

One goal for tomorrow:

Why:

- ☐ Make others happy
- ☐ Show love & support
- ☐ Challenge myself
- ☐ Feel good/have fun
- ☐ Complete overdue task
- ☐ Resolve something
- ☐ Make progress
- ☐ Relax

"Take the initiative. . . . Above all cooperate and don't hold back on one another or try to gain at the expense of another."
—BUCKMINSTER FULLER

WEEKEND

DATE: __/__/__

Success of the week:

Best experience of the week:

One treat planned for the weekend:

One inspiration/realization:

DATE: ___/___/___

"In order to succeed, we must first believe that we can." —**NIKOS KAZANTZAKIS**

One success I had today:

One redo I want:

One goal for tomorrow:

Why:

☐ Make others happy
☐ Show love & support
☐ Challenge myself
☐ Feel good/have fun
☐ Complete overdue task
☐ Resolve something
☐ Make progress
☐ Relax

TUESDAY

DATE: __/__/__

*" 'Fries or salad?' Sums up every adult decision
you have to make."* —**APARNA NANCHERLA**

One happiness today:

One screwup:

One intention for tomorrow:

Why:

- ☐ Make others happy
- ☐ Show love & support
- ☐ Challenge myself
- ☐ Feel good/have fun
- ☐ Complete overdue task
- ☐ Resolve something
- ☐ Make progress
- ☐ Relax

"There is only one corner of the universe you can be certain of improving, and that is yourself."
—**ALDOUS HUXLEY**

WEDNESDAY

DATE: ___/___/___

One success I had today:

One redo I want:

One goal for tomorrow:

Why:

- ☐ Make others happy
- ☐ Show love & support
- ☐ Challenge myself
- ☐ Feel good/have fun
- ☐ Complete overdue task
- ☐ Resolve something
- ☐ Make progress
- ☐ Relax

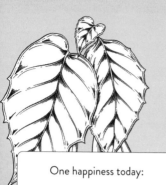

THURSDAY

DATE: __/__/__

*"We must let go of the life we have planned,
so as to accept the one that is waiting for us."*
—JOSEPH CAMPBELL

One happiness today:

One screwup:

One intention for tomorrow:

Why:

☐ Make others happy
☐ Show love & support
☐ Challenge myself
☐ Feel good/have fun
☐ Complete overdue task
☐ Resolve something
☐ Make progress
☐ Relax

DATE: ___/___/___

"No bird soars too high if he soars with his own wings." **—WILLIAM BLAKE**

One success I had today:

One redo I want:

One goal for tomorrow:

Why:

☐ Make others happy
☐ Show love & support
☐ Challenge myself
☐ Feel good/have fun
☐ Complete overdue task
☐ Resolve something
☐ Make progress
☐ Relax

DATE: __/__/__

"To read well, that is to read true books in a true spirit, is a noble exercise."
—HENRY DAVID THOREAU

Success of the week:

Best experience of the week:

One treat planned for the weekend:

One inspiration/realization:

"Either I will find a way, or I will make one."
—PHILIP SIDNEY

DATE: __/__/__

One happiness today:

One screwup:

One intention for tomorrow:

Why:

- ☐ Make others happy
- ☐ Show love & support
- ☐ Challenge myself
- ☐ Feel good/have fun
- ☐ Complete overdue task
- ☐ Resolve something
- ☐ Make progress
- ☐ Relax

TUESDAY

DATE: __/__/__

One success I had today:

One redo I want:

One goal for tomorrow:

Why:

- ☐ Make others happy
- ☐ Show love & support
- ☐ Challenge myself
- ☐ Feel good/have fun
- ☐ Complete overdue task
- ☐ Resolve something
- ☐ Make progress
- ☐ Relax

"Aim for the moon. If you miss, you may hit a star."
—W. CLEMENT STONE

One happiness today:

One screwup:

One intention for tomorrow:

Why:

☐ Make others happy
☐ Show love & support
☐ Challenge myself
☐ Feel good/have fun
☐ Complete overdue task
☐ Resolve something
☐ Make progress
☐ Relax

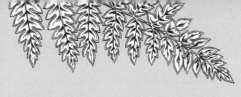

DATE: __/__/__

"My fake plants died because I did not pretend to water them." **—MITCH HEDBERG**

One success I had today:

One redo I want:

One goal for tomorrow:

Why:

- ☐ Make others happy
- ☐ Show love & support
- ☐ Challenge myself
- ☐ Feel good/have fun
- ☐ Complete overdue task
- ☐ Resolve something
- ☐ Make progress
- ☐ Relax

DATE: __/__/__

> *"You simply have to put one foot in front of the other and keep going. Put blinders on and plow right ahead."* **—GEORGE LUCAS**

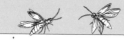

One happiness today:

One screwup:

One intention for tomorrow:

Why:

- [ ] Make others happy
- [ ] Show love & support
- [ ] Challenge myself
- [ ] Feel good/have fun
- [ ] Complete overdue task
- [ ] Resolve something
- [ ] Make progress
- [ ] Relax

"Nothing prepared me for being this awesome."
—BILL MURRAY

DATE: __/__/__

Success of the week:

Best experience of the week:

One treat planned for the weekend:

One inspiration/realization:

"Decide what you want, decide what you are willing to exchange for it. Establish your priorities and go to work." **–H. L. HUNT**

MONDAY

DATE: __/__/__

One success I had today:

One redo I want:

One goal for tomorrow:

Why:

☐ Make others happy
☐ Show love & support
☐ Challenge myself
☐ Feel good/have fun
☐ Complete overdue task
☐ Resolve something
☐ Make progress
☐ Relax

"Humor is the great thing, the saving thing. The minute it crops up, all our hardnesses yield, all our irritations and resentments flit away."
—MARK TWAIN

One happiness today:

One screwup:

One intention for tomorrow:

Why:

☐ Make others happy
☐ Show love & support
☐ Challenge myself
☐ Feel good/have fun
☐ Complete overdue task
☐ Resolve something
☐ Make progress
☐ Relax

WEDNESDAY

DATE: __/__/__

"You just can't beat the person who never gives up." **—BABE RUTH**

One success I had today:

One redo I want:

One goal for tomorrow:

Why:

☐ Make others happy
☐ Show love & support
☐ Challenge myself
☐ Feel good/have fun
☐ Complete overdue task
☐ Resolve something
☐ Make progress
☐ Relax

"Just because you're offended doesn't mean you're right." —**RICKY GERVAIS**

DATE: __/__/__

One happiness today:

One screwup:

One intention for tomorrow:

Why:

☐ Make others happy
☐ Show love & support
☐ Challenge myself
☐ Feel good/have fun
☐ Complete overdue task
☐ Resolve something
☐ Make progress
☐ Relax

DATE: __/__/__

"I do not fear men-at-arms; my way has been made plain before me." —**JOAN OF ARC**

One success I had today:

One redo I want:

One goal for tomorrow:

Why:

- ☐ Make others happy
- ☐ Show love & support
- ☐ Challenge myself
- ☐ Feel good/have fun
- ☐ Complete overdue task
- ☐ Resolve something
- ☐ Make progress
- ☐ Relax

A TIME TO REVIEW

DATE: __/__/__

What has changed for me?

What themes recurred over the year?

What do I now want to change?

Why:

- ☐ It was not serving me well
- ☐ It is not my business
- ☐ To grow stronger
- ☐ To be more loving
- ☐ To be more resilient
- ☐ To be more determined

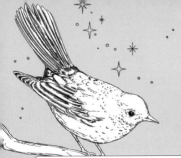

MONDAY

DATE: __/__/__

"You can never quit. Winners never quit, and quitters never win." —**ANONYMOUS**

One happiness today:

One screwup:

One intention for tomorrow:

Why:

☐ Make others happy
☐ Show love & support
☐ Challenge myself
☐ Feel good/have fun
☐ Complete overdue task
☐ Resolve something
☐ Make progress
☐ Relax

TUESDAY

"Confidence is 10 percent work and 90 percent delusion." **—TINA FEY**

DATE: __/__/__

One success I had today:

One redo I want:

One goal for tomorrow:

Why:

- ☐ Make others happy
- ☐ Show love & support
- ☐ Challenge myself
- ☐ Feel good/have fun
- ☐ Complete overdue task
- ☐ Resolve something
- ☐ Make progress
- ☐ Relax

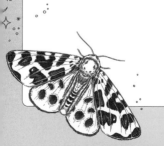

WEDNESDAY

"Without hard work, nothing grows but weeds."
—GORDON B. HINCKLEY

DATE: __/__/__

One happiness today:

One screwup:

One intention for tomorrow:

Why:

- [ ] Make others happy
- [ ] Show love & support
- [ ] Challenge myself
- [ ] Feel good/have fun
- [ ] Complete overdue task
- [ ] Resolve something
- [ ] Make progress
- [ ] Relax

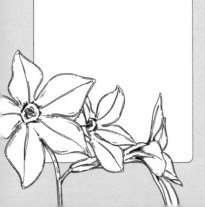

DATE: __/__/__

*"The streets of London have their map;
but our passions are uncharted. What are
you going to meet if you turn this corner?"*
—VIRGINIA WOOLF

One success I had today:

One redo I want:

One goal for tomorrow:

Why:

☐ Make others happy
☐ Show love & support
☐ Challenge myself
☐ Feel good/have fun
☐ Complete overdue task
☐ Resolve something
☐ Make progress
☐ Relax

FRIDAY

DATE: __/__/__

"I really believe that everyone has a talent, ability, or skill that he can mine to support himself and to succeed in life." **—DEAN KOONTZ**

One happiness today:

One screwup:

One intention for tomorrow:

Why:

- ☐ Make others happy
- ☐ Show love & support
- ☐ Challenge myself
- ☐ Feel good/have fun
- ☐ Complete overdue task
- ☐ Resolve something
- ☐ Make progress
- ☐ Relax

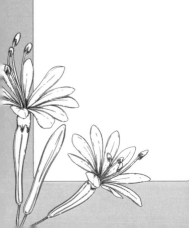

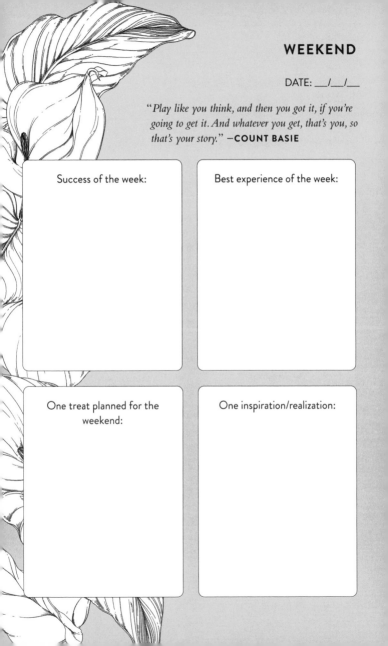

WEEKEND

DATE: __/__/__

"Play like you think, and then you got it, if you're going to get it. And whatever you get, that's you, so that's your story." —**COUNT BASIE**

Success of the week:

Best experience of the week:

One treat planned for the weekend:

One inspiration/realization:

DATE: ___/___/___

"Opportunity does not knock, it presents itself when you beat down the door."
—KYLE CHANDLER

One success I had today:

One redo I want:

One goal for tomorrow:

Why:

- ☐ Make others happy
- ☐ Show love & support
- ☐ Challenge myself
- ☐ Feel good/have fun
- ☐ Complete overdue task
- ☐ Resolve something
- ☐ Make progress
- ☐ Relax

*"Sometimes I'm really funny, sometimes I'm quiet,
sometimes I'm shy, but I'm constantly changing."*
—ELLE KING

DATE: __/__/__

One happiness today:

One screwup:

One intention for tomorrow:

Why:

- ☐ Make others happy
- ☐ Show love & support
- ☐ Challenge myself
- ☐ Feel good/have fun
- ☐ Complete overdue task
- ☐ Resolve something
- ☐ Make progress
- ☐ Relax

"I attribute my success to this—I never gave or took any excuse."
—FLORENCE NIGHTINGALE

DATE: __/__/__

One success I had today:

One redo I want:

One goal for tomorrow:

Why:

- ☐ Make others happy
- ☐ Show love & support
- ☐ Challenge myself
- ☐ Feel good/have fun
- ☐ Complete overdue task
- ☐ Resolve something
- ☐ Make progress
- ☐ Relax

DATE: __/__/__

"An education isn't how much you have committed to memory. . . . It's knowing how to use the information once you get it."
—WILLIAM FEATHER

One happiness today:

One screwup:

One intention for tomorrow:

Why:

- ☐ Make others happy
- ☐ Show love & support
- ☐ Challenge myself
- ☐ Feel good/have fun
- ☐ Complete overdue task
- ☐ Resolve something
- ☐ Make progress
- ☐ Relax

"You will never win if you never begin."
—HELEN ROWLAND

One success I had today:

One redo I want:

One goal for tomorrow:

Why:

- [ ] Make others happy
- [ ] Show love & support
- [ ] Challenge myself
- [ ] Feel good/have fun
- [ ] Complete overdue task
- [ ] Resolve something
- [ ] Make progress
- [ ] Relax

"More and more as we come closer and closer in touch with nature and its teachings are we able to see the Divine." **—GEORGE WASHINGTON CARVER**

Success of the week:

Best experience of the week:

One treat planned for the weekend:

One inspiration/realization:

"Never retreat. Never explain. Get it done and let them howl." —**BENJAMIN JOWETT**

DATE: __/__/__

One happiness today:

One screwup:

One intention for tomorrow:

Why:

- [ ] Make others happy
- [ ] Show love & support
- [ ] Challenge myself
- [ ] Feel good/have fun
- [ ] Complete overdue task
- [ ] Resolve something
- [ ] Make progress
- [ ] Relax

"Censorship works by flooding you with immense amounts of misinformation, of irrelevant information, of funny cat videos, until you're just unable to focus." **—YUVAL NOAH HARARI**

One success I had today:

One redo I want:

One goal for tomorrow:

Why:

- ☐ Make others happy
- ☐ Show love & support
- ☐ Challenge myself
- ☐ Feel good/have fun
- ☐ Complete overdue task
- ☐ Resolve something
- ☐ Make progress
- ☐ Relax

DATE: __/__/__

"Discipline for me has always been the foundation which leaves me free to fly." —**JULIE ANDREWS**

One happiness today:

One screwup:

One intention for tomorrow:

Why:

☐ Make others happy
☐ Show love & support
☐ Challenge myself
☐ Feel good/have fun
☐ Complete overdue task
☐ Resolve something
☐ Make progress
☐ Relax

"For myself I am an optimist—it does not seem to be much use being anything else."
—WINSTON CHURCHILL

One success I had today:

One redo I want:

One goal for tomorrow:

Why:

- ☐ Make others happy
- ☐ Show love & support
- ☐ Challenge myself
- ☐ Feel good/have fun
- ☐ Complete overdue task
- ☐ Resolve something
- ☐ Make progress
- ☐ Relax

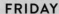

"The ultimate aim of the ego is not to see something, but to be something."
—MUHAMMAD IQBAL

DATE: __/__/__

One happiness today:

One screwup:

One intention for tomorrow:

Why:

☐ Make others happy
☐ Show love & support
☐ Challenge myself
☐ Feel good/have fun
☐ Complete overdue task
☐ Resolve something
☐ Make progress
☐ Relax

"Two wrongs don't make a right, but they make a good excuse." —**THOMAS SZASZ**

DATE: __/__/__

Success of the week:

Best experience of the week:

One treat planned for the weekend:

One inspiration/realization:

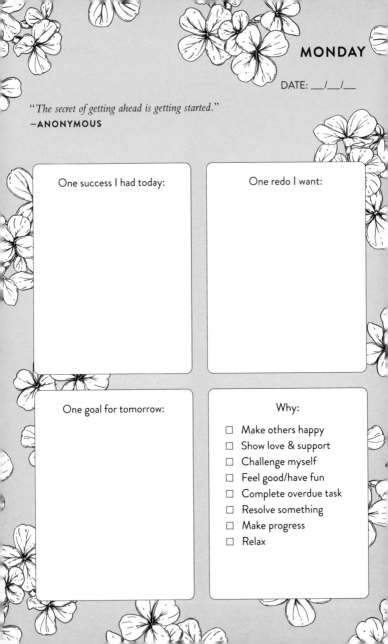

MONDAY

DATE: __/__/__

"The secret of getting ahead is getting started."
—ANONYMOUS

One success I had today:

One redo I want:

One goal for tomorrow:

Why:

☐ Make others happy
☐ Show love & support
☐ Challenge myself
☐ Feel good/have fun
☐ Complete overdue task
☐ Resolve something
☐ Make progress
☐ Relax

"Mend when thou canst; be better at thy leisure."
—SHAKESPEARE

One happiness today:

One screwup:

One intention for tomorrow:

Why:

- ☐ Make others happy
- ☐ Show love & support
- ☐ Challenge myself
- ☐ Feel good/have fun
- ☐ Complete overdue task
- ☐ Resolve something
- ☐ Make progress
- ☐ Relax

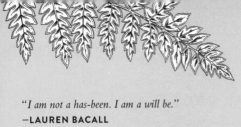

WEDNESDAY

DATE: ___/___/___

"I am not a has-been. I am a will be."
—LAUREN BACALL

One success I had today:

One redo I want:

One goal for tomorrow:

Why:

☐ Make others happy
☐ Show love & support
☐ Challenge myself
☐ Feel good/have fun
☐ Complete overdue task
☐ Resolve something
☐ Make progress
☐ Relax

THURSDAY

"Meditation is the soul's perspective glass."
—OWEN FELTHAM

DATE: __/__/__

One happiness today:

One screwup:

One intention for tomorrow:

Why:

- ☐ Make others happy
- ☐ Show love & support
- ☐ Challenge myself
- ☐ Feel good/have fun
- ☐ Complete overdue task
- ☐ Resolve something
- ☐ Make progress
- ☐ Relax

FRIDAY

"If you're going through hell, keep going."
—ANONYMOUS

DATE: __/__/__

One success I had today:

One redo I want:

One goal for tomorrow:

Why:

- ☐ Make others happy
- ☐ Show love & support
- ☐ Challenge myself
- ☐ Feel good/have fun
- ☐ Complete overdue task
- ☐ Resolve something
- ☐ Make progress
- ☐ Relax

"What does it cost to add a smile?"
—JEAN DE LA BRUYÈRE

DATE: __/__/__

Success of the week:

Best experience of the week:

One treat planned for the weekend:

One inspiration/realization:

MONDAY

DATE: __/__/__

"Well done is better than well said."
—BENJAMIN FRANKLIN

One happiness today:

One screwup:

One intention for tomorrow:

Why:

- ☐ Make others happy
- ☐ Show love & support
- ☐ Challenge myself
- ☐ Feel good/have fun
- ☐ Complete overdue task
- ☐ Resolve something
- ☐ Make progress
- ☐ Relax

"The difference between perseverance and obstinacy is that one comes from a strong will, and the other from a strong won't."
—HENRY WARD BEECHER

One success I had today:

One redo I want:

One goal for tomorrow:

Why:

- ☐ Make others happy
- ☐ Show love & support
- ☐ Challenge myself
- ☐ Feel good/have fun
- ☐ Complete overdue task
- ☐ Resolve something
- ☐ Make progress
- ☐ Relax

"Be miserable. Or motivate yourself. Whatever has to be done, it's always your choice."
—WAYNE DYER

DATE: ___/___/___

One happiness today:

One screwup:

One intention for tomorrow:

Why:

- [ ] Make others happy
- [ ] Show love & support
- [ ] Challenge myself
- [ ] Feel good/have fun
- [ ] Complete overdue task
- [ ] Resolve something
- [ ] Make progress
- [ ] Relax

THURSDAY

DATE: __/__/__

"To sleep! perchance to dream; ay, there's the rub." —**SHAKESPEARE**

One success I had today:

One redo I want:

One goal for tomorrow:

Why:

- ☐ Make others happy
- ☐ Show love & support
- ☐ Challenge myself
- ☐ Feel good/have fun
- ☐ Complete overdue task
- ☐ Resolve something
- ☐ Make progress
- ☐ Relax

FRIDAY

DATE: __/__/__

"By failing to prepare, you are preparing to fail."
—BENJAMIN FRANKLIN

One happiness today:

One screwup:

One intention for tomorrow:

Why:

- ☐ Make others happy
- ☐ Show love & support
- ☐ Challenge myself
- ☐ Feel good/have fun
- ☐ Complete overdue task
- ☐ Resolve something
- ☐ Make progress
- ☐ Relax

WEEKEND

DATE: __/__/__

"Next time you have a thought . . . let it go." —RON WHITE

Success of the week:

Best experience of the week:

One treat planned for the weekend:

One inspiration/realization:

DATE: ___/___/___

"It does not matter how slowly you go as long as you do not stop." **—CONFUCIUS**

One happiness today:

One screwup:

One intention for tomorrow:

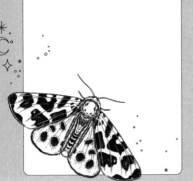

Why:

☐ Make others happy
☐ Show love & support
☐ Challenge myself
☐ Feel good/have fun
☐ Complete overdue task
☐ Resolve something
☐ Make progress
☐ Relax

TUESDAY

DATE: __/__/__

"What, then, shall we do? . . . What else, indeed,
than devote ourselves to the care of our souls."
—BASIL OF CAESAREA

One success I had today:

One redo I want:

One goal for tomorrow:

Why:

- ☐ Make others happy
- ☐ Show love & support
- ☐ Challenge myself
- ☐ Feel good/have fun
- ☐ Complete overdue task
- ☐ Resolve something
- ☐ Make progress
- ☐ Relax

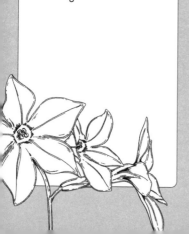

WEDNESDAY

DATE: __/__/__

"Keep your eyes on the stars, and your feet on the ground." **—THEODORE ROOSEVELT**

One happiness today:

One screwup:

One intention for tomorrow:

Why:

- ☐ Make others happy
- ☐ Show love & support
- ☐ Challenge myself
- ☐ Feel good/have fun
- ☐ Complete overdue task
- ☐ Resolve something
- ☐ Make progress
- ☐ Relax

DATE: __/__/__

"Wisdom is born of meditation; without meditation, wisdom is lost."
—**GAUTAMA BUDDHA**

One success I had today:

One redo I want:

One goal for tomorrow:

Why:

☐ Make others happy
☐ Show love & support
☐ Challenge myself
☐ Feel good/have fun
☐ Complete overdue task
☐ Resolve something
☐ Make progress
☐ Relax

"Act as if what you do makes a difference. It does." —**WILLIAM JAMES**

DATE: ___/___/___

One happiness today:

One screwup:

One intention for tomorrow:

Why:

- ☐ Make others happy
- ☐ Show love & support
- ☐ Challenge myself
- ☐ Feel good/have fun
- ☐ Complete overdue task
- ☐ Resolve something
- ☐ Make progress
- ☐ Relax

"Whenever you are able to observe your mind, you are no longer trapped in it." **—ECKHART TOLLE**

DATE: __/__/__

Success of the week:

Best experience of the week:

One treat planned for the weekend:

One inspiration/realization:

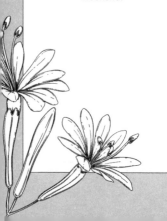

"You are here to enrich the world, and you impoverish yourself if you forget the errand."
—WOODROW WILSON

One success I had today:

One redo I want:

One goal for tomorrow:

Why:

☐ Make others happy
☐ Show love & support
☐ Challenge myself
☐ Feel good/have fun
☐ Complete overdue task
☐ Resolve something
☐ Make progress
☐ Relax

"Life is a long lesson in humility." —**J. M. BARRIE**

One happiness today:

One screwup:

One intention for tomorrow:

Why:

- ☐ Make others happy
- ☐ Show love & support
- ☐ Challenge myself
- ☐ Feel good/have fun
- ☐ Complete overdue task
- ☐ Resolve something
- ☐ Make progress
- ☐ Relax

WEDNESDAY

DATE: ___/___/___

"They can because they think they can."
—VIRGIL

One success I had today:

One redo I want:

One goal for tomorrow:

Why:

- [ ] Make others happy
- [ ] Show love & support
- [ ] Challenge myself
- [ ] Feel good/have fun
- [ ] Complete overdue task
- [ ] Resolve something
- [ ] Make progress
- [ ] Relax

"Instant gratification takes too long."
—CARRIE FISHER

DATE: __/__/__

One happiness today:

One screwup:

One intention for tomorrow:

Why:

☐ Make others happy
☐ Show love & support
☐ Challenge myself
☐ Feel good/have fun
☐ Complete overdue task
☐ Resolve something
☐ Make progress
☐ Relax

DATE: ___/___/___

"One way to keep momentum going is to have constantly greater goals." —**MICHAEL KORDA**

One success I had today:

One redo I want:

One goal for tomorrow:

Why:

- ☐ Make others happy
- ☐ Show love & support
- ☐ Challenge myself
- ☐ Feel good/have fun
- ☐ Complete overdue task
- ☐ Resolve something
- ☐ Make progress
- ☐ Relax

"He was like a cock who thought the sun had risen to hear him crow." —**GEORGE ELIOT**

Success of the week:

Best experience of the week:

One treat planned for the weekend:

One inspiration/realization:

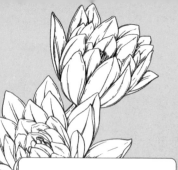

MONDAY

DATE: __/__/__

"Never complain and never explain."
—BENJAMIN DISRAELI

One success I had today:

One redo I want:

One goal for tomorrow:

Why:

- ☐ Make others happy
- ☐ Show love & support
- ☐ Challenge myself
- ☐ Feel good/have fun
- ☐ Complete overdue task
- ☐ Resolve something
- ☐ Make progress
- ☐ Relax

"An optimist is a fellow who believes a housefly is looking for a way to get out."
—GEORGE JEAN NATHAN

One happiness today:

One screwup:

One intention for tomorrow:

Why:

- ☐ Make others happy
- ☐ Show love & support
- ☐ Challenge myself
- ☐ Feel good/have fun
- ☐ Complete overdue task
- ☐ Resolve something
- ☐ Make progress
- ☐ Relax

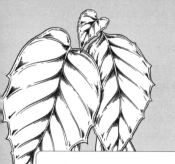

WEDNESDAY

DATE: __/__/__

"A journey of a thousand miles starts with a single step." **—LAO TZU**

One success I had today:

One redo I want:

One goal for tomorrow:

Why:

- ☐ Make others happy
- ☐ Show love & support
- ☐ Challenge myself
- ☐ Feel good/have fun
- ☐ Complete overdue task
- ☐ Resolve something
- ☐ Make progress
- ☐ Relax

"Every cloud has a silver lining."
—ANONYMOUS

DATE: __/__/__

One happiness today:

One screwup:

One intention for tomorrow:

Why:

☐ Make others happy
☐ Show love & support
☐ Challenge myself
☐ Feel good/have fun
☐ Complete overdue task
☐ Resolve something
☐ Make progress
☐ Relax

"Isn't it a pleasure to study and practice what you have learned?" —**CONFUCIUS**

DATE: __/__/__

One success I had today:

One redo I want:

One goal for tomorrow:

Why:

- ☐ Make others happy
- ☐ Show love & support
- ☐ Challenge myself
- ☐ Feel good/have fun
- ☐ Complete overdue task
- ☐ Resolve something
- ☐ Make progress
- ☐ Relax

"I'm an optimist, but an optimist who carries a raincoat." —**HAROLD WILSON**

DATE: __/__/__

Success of the week:

Best experience of the week:

One treat planned for the weekend:

One inspiration/realization:

"Don't think, just do." **—HORACE**

DATE: __/__/__

One happiness today:

One screwup:

One intention for tomorrow:

Why:

- [ ] Make others happy
- [ ] Show love & support
- [ ] Challenge myself
- [ ] Feel good/have fun
- [ ] Complete overdue task
- [ ] Resolve something
- [ ] Make progress
- [ ] Relax

"Look up and not down; look forward and not back; look out and not in; lend a hand."
—EDWARD EVERETT HALE

DATE: ___/___/___

One success I had today:

One redo I want:

One goal for tomorrow:

Why:

- ☐ Make others happy
- ☐ Show love & support
- ☐ Challenge myself
- ☐ Feel good/have fun
- ☐ Complete overdue task
- ☐ Resolve something
- ☐ Make progress
- ☐ Relax

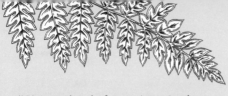

"Setting goals is the first step in turning the invisible into the visible." **—TONY ROBBINS**

One happiness today:

One screwup:

One intention for tomorrow:

Why:

- ☐ Make others happy
- ☐ Show love & support
- ☐ Challenge myself
- ☐ Feel good/have fun
- ☐ Complete overdue task
- ☐ Resolve something
- ☐ Make progress
- ☐ Relax

THURSDAY

DATE: __/__/__

"I must learn to brook being happier than I deserve." **–JANE AUSTEN**

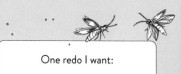

One success I had today:

One redo I want:

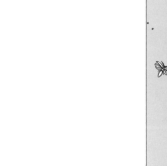

One goal for tomorrow:

Why:

- ☐ Make others happy
- ☐ Show love & support
- ☐ Challenge myself
- ☐ Feel good/have fun
- ☐ Complete overdue task
- ☐ Resolve something
- ☐ Make progress
- ☐ Relax

"If you think you can do it, you can."
—JOHN BURROUGHS

DATE: __/__/__

One happiness today:

One screwup:

One intention for tomorrow:

Why:

- ☐ Make others happy
- ☐ Show love & support
- ☐ Challenge myself
- ☐ Feel good/have fun
- ☐ Complete overdue task
- ☐ Resolve something
- ☐ Make progress
- ☐ Relax

Success of the week:

Best experience of the week:

One treat planned for the weekend:

One inspiration/realization:

MONDAY

"You are never too old to set another goal or to dream a new dream." **—LES BROWN**

DATE: __/__/__

One success I had today:

One redo I want:

One goal for tomorrow:

Why:

- ☐ Make others happy
- ☐ Show love & support
- ☐ Challenge myself
- ☐ Feel good/have fun
- ☐ Complete overdue task
- ☐ Resolve something
- ☐ Make progress
- ☐ Relax

"If you can't make it better, you can laugh at it."
—ERMA BOMBECK

DATE: ___/___/___

One happiness today:

One screwup:

One intention for tomorrow:

Why:

☐ Make others happy
☐ Show love & support
☐ Challenge myself
☐ Feel good/have fun
☐ Complete overdue task
☐ Resolve something
☐ Make progress
☐ Relax

WEDNESDAY

DATE: __/__/__

"The people who influence you are the people who believe in you." —**HENRY DRUMMOND**

One success I had today:

One redo I want:

One goal for tomorrow:

Why:
- ☐ Make others happy
- ☐ Show love & support
- ☐ Challenge myself
- ☐ Feel good/have fun
- ☐ Complete overdue task
- ☐ Resolve something
- ☐ Make progress
- ☐ Relax

"Success always demands a greater effort."
—WINSTON CHURCHILL

DATE: __/__/__

One happiness today:

One screwup:

One intention for tomorrow:

Why:

- ☐ Make others happy
- ☐ Show love & support
- ☐ Challenge myself
- ☐ Feel good/have fun
- ☐ Complete overdue task
- ☐ Resolve something
- ☐ Make progress
- ☐ Relax

DATE: __/__/__

"Optimism is the faith that leads to achievement. Nothing can be done without hope and confidence." —**HELEN KELLER**

One success I had today:

One redo I want:

One goal for tomorrow:

Why:

☐ Make others happy
☐ Show love & support
☐ Challenge myself
☐ Feel good/have fun
☐ Complete overdue task
☐ Resolve something
☐ Make progress
☐ Relax

WEEKEND

DATE: __/__/__

"Condition, circumstance, is not the thing;
Bliss is the same in subject or in king."
—ALEXANDER POPE

Success of the week:

Best experience of the week:

One treat planned for the weekend:

One inspiration/realization:

DATE: __/__/__

"No matter how many goals you have achieved, you must set your sights on a higher one."
—JESSICA SAVITCH

One success I had today:

One redo I want:

One goal for tomorrow:

Why:

- ☐ Make others happy
- ☐ Show love & support
- ☐ Challenge myself
- ☐ Feel good/have fun
- ☐ Complete overdue task
- ☐ Resolve something
- ☐ Make progress
- ☐ Relax

"An attitude is almost like a muscle. You can choose to have a good one. Find ways to exercise it and make it grow." **—JERRY S. BEALL**

DATE: __/__/__

One happiness today:

One screwup:

One intention for tomorrow:

Why:

☐ Make others happy
☐ Show love & support
☐ Challenge myself
☐ Feel good/have fun
☐ Complete overdue task
☐ Resolve something
☐ Make progress
☐ Relax

*"Do not wait; the time will never be 'just right.'
Start where you stand, and work with whatever
tools you may have at your command, and better
tools will be found as you go along."*
—GEORGE HERBERT

One success I had today:

One redo I want:

One goal for tomorrow:

Why:

☐ Make others happy
☐ Show love & support
☐ Challenge myself
☐ Feel good/have fun
☐ Complete overdue task
☐ Resolve something
☐ Make progress
☐ Relax

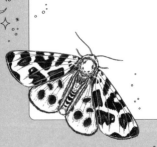

THURSDAY

DATE: __/__/__

"Do not worry about avoiding temptation.
As you grow older it will avoid you."
—JOEY ADAMS

One happiness today:

One screwup:

One intention for tomorrow:

Why:

- ☐ Make others happy
- ☐ Show love & support
- ☐ Challenge myself
- ☐ Feel good/have fun
- ☐ Complete overdue task
- ☐ Resolve something
- ☐ Make progress
- ☐ Relax

FRIDAY

"The hardships that I encountered in the past will help me succeed in the future."
—PHILIP EMEAGWALI

DATE: __/__/__

One success I had today:

One redo I want:

One goal for tomorrow:

Why:

- ☐ Make others happy
- ☐ Show love & support
- ☐ Challenge myself
- ☐ Feel good/have fun
- ☐ Complete overdue task
- ☐ Resolve something
- ☐ Make progress
- ☐ Relax

WEEKEND

DATE: __/__/__

"We all need joy, and we can all receive joy in only one way, by adding to the joy of others."
—EKNATH EASWARAN

Success of the week:

Best experience of the week:

One treat planned for the weekend:

One inspiration/realization:

MONDAY

DATE: __/__/__

"Motivation will almost always beat mere talent."
—NORMAN RALPH AUGUSTINE

One happiness today:

One screwup:

One intention for tomorrow:

Why:

- ☐ Make others happy
- ☐ Show love & support
- ☐ Challenge myself
- ☐ Feel good/have fun
- ☐ Complete overdue task
- ☐ Resolve something
- ☐ Make progress
- ☐ Relax

"Perfect tranquility within consists in the good ordering of the mind, the realm of your own."
—MARCUS AURELIUS

DATE: __/__/__

One success I had today:

One redo I want:

One goal for tomorrow:

Why:

☐ Make others happy
☐ Show love & support
☐ Challenge myself
☐ Feel good/have fun
☐ Complete overdue task
☐ Resolve something
☐ Make progress
☐ Relax

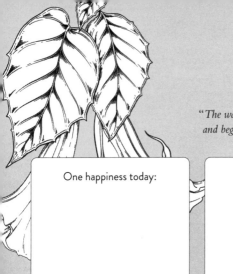

"The way to get started is to quit talking and begin doing." —**WALT DISNEY**

One happiness today:

One screwup:

One intention for tomorrow:

Why:

- ☐ Make others happy
- ☐ Show love & support
- ☐ Challenge myself
- ☐ Feel good/have fun
- ☐ Complete overdue task
- ☐ Resolve something
- ☐ Make progress
- ☐ Relax

"I have a new philosophy. I'm only going to dread one day at a time." —**CHARLES M. SCHULZ**

DATE: __/__/__

One success I had today:

One redo I want:

One goal for tomorrow:

Why:

- ☐ Make others happy
- ☐ Show love & support
- ☐ Challenge myself
- ☐ Feel good/have fun
- ☐ Complete overdue task
- ☐ Resolve something
- ☐ Make progress
- ☐ Relax

"There is no passion to be found playing small—in settling for a life that is less than the one you are capable of living." **—NELSON MANDELA**

DATE: __/__/__

One happiness today:

One screwup:

One intention for tomorrow:

Why:

- ☐ Make others happy
- ☐ Show love & support
- ☐ Challenge myself
- ☐ Feel good/have fun
- ☐ Complete overdue task
- ☐ Resolve something
- ☐ Make progress
- ☐ Relax

"The only way to have a good friend is to be one."
—RALPH WALDO EMERSON

DATE: __/__/__

Success of the week:

Best experience of the week:

One treat planned for the weekend:

One inspiration/realization:

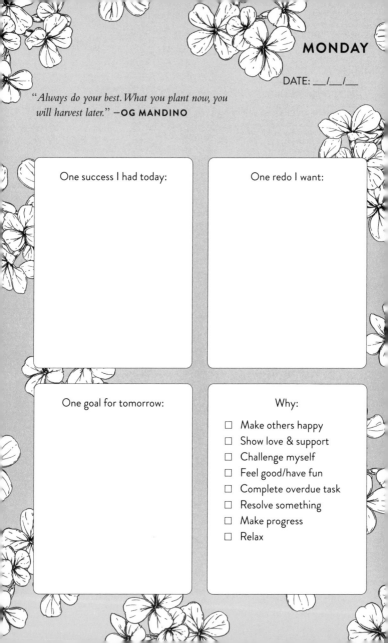

MONDAY

DATE: ___/___/___

"Always do your best. What you plant now, you will harvest later." —**OG MANDINO**

One success I had today:

One redo I want:

One goal for tomorrow:

Why:

- ☐ Make others happy
- ☐ Show love & support
- ☐ Challenge myself
- ☐ Feel good/have fun
- ☐ Complete overdue task
- ☐ Resolve something
- ☐ Make progress
- ☐ Relax

DATE: __/__/__

"Art . . . is the authentic expression of any and all individuality." **—JOHN DEWEY**

One happiness today:

One screwup:

One intention for tomorrow:

Why:

☐ Make others happy
☐ Show love & support
☐ Challenge myself
☐ Feel good/have fun
☐ Complete overdue task
☐ Resolve something
☐ Make progress
☐ Relax

"Our greatest weakness lies in giving up. The most certain way to succeed is always to try just one more time." **—THOMAS A. EDISON**

WEDNESDAY

DATE: __/__/__

One success I had today:

One redo I want:

One goal for tomorrow:

Why:

- ☐ Make others happy
- ☐ Show love & support
- ☐ Challenge myself
- ☐ Feel good/have fun
- ☐ Complete overdue task
- ☐ Resolve something
- ☐ Make progress
- ☐ Relax

THURSDAY

DATE: __/__/__

One happiness today:

One screwup:

One intention for tomorrow:

Why:

☐ Make others happy
☐ Show love & support
☐ Challenge myself
☐ Feel good/have fun
☐ Complete overdue task
☐ Resolve something
☐ Make progress
☐ Relax

"To begin, begin." —**WILLIAM WORDSWORTH**

DATE: __/__/__

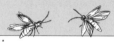

One success I had today:

One redo I want:

One goal for tomorrow:

Why:

- ☐ Make others happy
- ☐ Show love & support
- ☐ Challenge myself
- ☐ Feel good/have fun
- ☐ Complete overdue task
- ☐ Resolve something
- ☐ Make progress
- ☐ Relax

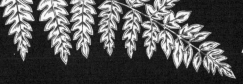

A TIME TO REVIEW

DATE: __/__/__

What has changed for me?

What themes recurred over the year?

What do I now want to change?

Why:

- ☐ It was not serving me well
- ☐ It is not my business
- ☐ To grow stronger
- ☐ To be more loving
- ☐ To be more resilient
- ☐ To be more determined

"There is always room at the top."
—DANIEL WEBSTER

DATE: __/__/__

One happiness today:

One screwup:

One intention for tomorrow:

Why:

- ☐ Make others happy
- ☐ Show love & support
- ☐ Challenge myself
- ☐ Feel good/have fun
- ☐ Complete overdue task
- ☐ Resolve something
- ☐ Make progress
- ☐ Relax

One success I had today:

One redo I want:

One goal for tomorrow:

Why:

☐ Make others happy
☐ Show love & support
☐ Challenge myself
☐ Feel good/have fun
☐ Complete overdue task
☐ Resolve something
☐ Make progress
☐ Relax

"Follow your inner moonlight; don't hide the madness." —**ALLEN GINSBERG**

DATE: __/__/__

One happiness today:

One screwup:

One intention for tomorrow:

Why:

- ☐ Make others happy
- ☐ Show love & support
- ☐ Challenge myself
- ☐ Feel good/have fun
- ☐ Complete overdue task
- ☐ Resolve something
- ☐ Make progress
- ☐ Relax

"We turn not older with years, but newer every day." —**EMILY DICKINSON**

One success I had today:

One redo I want:

One goal for tomorrow:

Why:

- ☐ Make others happy
- ☐ Show love & support
- ☐ Challenge myself
- ☐ Feel good/have fun
- ☐ Complete overdue task
- ☐ Resolve something
- ☐ Make progress
- ☐ Relax

"Either you run the day, or the day runs you."
—JIM ROHN

DATE: __/__/__

One happiness today:

One screwup:

One intention for tomorrow:

Why:

- ☐ Make others happy
- ☐ Show love & support
- ☐ Challenge myself
- ☐ Feel good/have fun
- ☐ Complete overdue task
- ☐ Resolve something
- ☐ Make progress
- ☐ Relax

WEEKEND

DATE: __/__/__

"The nature of genius is to provide idiots with ideas twenty years later." —**LOUIS ARAGON**

Success of the week:

Best experience of the week:

One treat planned for the weekend:

One inspiration/realization:

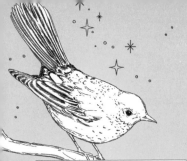

"Go for it now. The future is promised to no one." —**WAYNE DYER**

One happiness today:

One screwup:

One intention for tomorrow:

Why:

- ☐ Make others happy
- ☐ Show love & support
- ☐ Challenge myself
- ☐ Feel good/have fun
- ☐ Complete overdue task
- ☐ Resolve something
- ☐ Make progress
- ☐ Relax

TUESDAY

DATE: __/__/__

"If the shoe doesn't fit, must we change the foot?" —**GLORIA STEINEM**

One success I had today:

One redo I want:

One goal for tomorrow:

Why:

- ☐ Make others happy
- ☐ Show love & support
- ☐ Challenge myself
- ☐ Feel good/have fun
- ☐ Complete overdue task
- ☐ Resolve something
- ☐ Make progress
- ☐ Relax

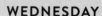

WEDNESDAY

"Step by step and the thing is done."
—CHARLES ATLAS

DATE: __/__/__

One happiness today:

One screwup:

One intention for tomorrow:

Why:

- ☐ Make others happy
- ☐ Show love & support
- ☐ Challenge myself
- ☐ Feel good/have fun
- ☐ Complete overdue task
- ☐ Resolve something
- ☐ Make progress
- ☐ Relax

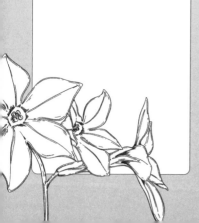

DATE: ___/___/___

"We have all a better guide in ourselves, if we would attend to it, than any other person can be."
—JANE AUSTEN

One success I had today:

One redo I want:

One goal for tomorrow:

Why:

- ☐ Make others happy
- ☐ Show love & support
- ☐ Challenge myself
- ☐ Feel good/have fun
- ☐ Complete overdue task
- ☐ Resolve something
- ☐ Make progress
- ☐ Relax

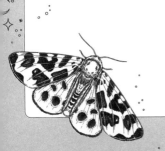

*"There is progress whether ye are going
forward or backward! The thing is to move!"*
—EDGAR CAYCE

DATE: __/__/__

One happiness today:

One screwup:

One intention for tomorrow

Why:

- ☐ Make others happy
- ☐ Show love & support
- ☐ Challenge myself
- ☐ Feel good/have fun
- ☐ Complete overdue task
- ☐ Resolve something
- ☐ Make progress
- ☐ Relax

DATE: __/__/__

"Each friend represents a world in us, a world possibly not born until they arrive, and it is only by this meeting that a new world is born."
—ANAÏS NIN

Success of the week:

Best experience of the week:

One treat planned for the weekend:

One inspiration/realization:

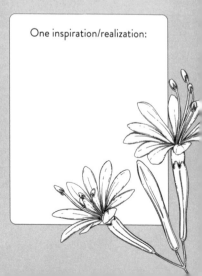

DATE: __/__/__

"He conquers who endures." **—PERSIUS**

One success I had today:

One redo I want:

One goal for tomorrow:

Why:

- ☐ Make others happy
- ☐ Show love & support
- ☐ Challenge myself
- ☐ Feel good/have fun
- ☐ Complete overdue task
- ☐ Resolve something
- ☐ Make progress
- ☐ Relax

"When we ask for advice, we are usually looking for an accomplice." —**SAUL BELLOW**

DATE: ___/___/___

One happiness today:

One screwup:

One intention for tomorrow:

Why:

- ☐ Make others happy
- ☐ Show love & support
- ☐ Challenge myself
- ☐ Feel good/have fun
- ☐ Complete overdue task
- ☐ Resolve something
- ☐ Make progress
- ☐ Relax

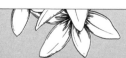

WEDNESDAY

DATE: ___/___/___

"You never know what motivates you."
—CICELY TYSON

One success I had today:

One redo I want:

One goal for tomorrow:

Why:

- ☐ Make others happy
- ☐ Show love & support
- ☐ Challenge myself
- ☐ Feel good/have fun
- ☐ Complete overdue task
- ☐ Resolve something
- ☐ Make progress
- ☐ Relax

"Vulnerability is the birthplace of love, belonging, joy, courage, empathy, and creativity."
—BRENÉ BROWN

DATE: __/__/__

One happiness today:

One screwup:

One intention for tomorrow:

Why:

- ☐ Make others happy
- ☐ Show love & support
- ☐ Challenge myself
- ☐ Feel good/have fun
- ☐ Complete overdue task
- ☐ Resolve something
- ☐ Make progress
- ☐ Relax

DATE: __/__/__

"A creative man is motivated by the desire to achieve, not by the desire to beat others."
—AYN RAND

One success I had today:

One redo I want:

One goal for tomorrow:

Why:

- ☐ Make others happy
- ☐ Show love & support
- ☐ Challenge myself
- ☐ Feel good/have fun
- ☐ Complete overdue task
- ☐ Resolve something
- ☐ Make progress
- ☐ Relax

"*I don't deserve any credit for turning the other cheek as my tongue is always in it.*"
—FLANNERY O'CONNOR

DATE: __/__/__

Success of the week:

Best experience of the week:

One treat planned for the weekend:

One inspiration/realization:

DATE: __/__/__

"Always desire to learn something useful."
—SOPHOCLES

One success I had today:

One redo I want:

One goal for tomorrow:

Why:

☐ Make others happy
☐ Show love & support
☐ Challenge myself
☐ Feel good/have fun
☐ Complete overdue task
☐ Resolve something
☐ Make progress
☐ Relax

"Loyalty to petrified opinions never yet broke a chain or freed a human soul in this world— and never will." **–MARK TWAIN**

One happiness today:

One screwup:

One intention for tomorrow:

Why:

- ☐ Make others happy
- ☐ Show love & support
- ☐ Challenge myself
- ☐ Feel good/have fun
- ☐ Complete overdue task
- ☐ Resolve something
- ☐ Make progress
- ☐ Relax

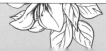

WEDNESDAY

DATE: __/__/__

"The most effective way to do it, is to do it."
—AMELIA EARHART

One success I had today:

One redo I want:

One goal for tomorrow:

Why:

- ☐ Make others happy
- ☐ Show love & support
- ☐ Challenge myself
- ☐ Feel good/have fun
- ☐ Complete overdue task
- ☐ Resolve something
- ☐ Make progress
- ☐ Relax

"To know oneself, one should assert oneself."
—ALBERT CAMUS

DATE: __/__/__

One happiness today:

One screwup:

One intention for tomorrow:

Why:

- ☐ Make others happy
- ☐ Show love & support
- ☐ Challenge myself
- ☐ Feel good/have fun
- ☐ Complete overdue task
- ☐ Resolve something
- ☐ Make progress
- ☐ Relax

DATE: ___/___/___

"What you get by achieving your goals is not as important as what you become by achieving your goals." **—ZIG ZIGLER**

One success I had today:

One redo I want:

One goal for tomorrow:

Why:

☐ Make others happy
☐ Show love & support
☐ Challenge myself
☐ Feel good/have fun
☐ Complete overdue task
☐ Resolve something
☐ Make progress
☐ Relax

"Love is a great beautifier."
—LOUISA MAY ALCOTT

DATE: __/__/__

Success of the week:

Best experience of the week:

One treat planned for the weekend:

One inspiration/realization:

DATE: __/__/__

"Small deeds done are better than great deeds planned." —**PETER MARSHALL**

One happiness today:

One screwup:

One intention for tomorrow:

Why:

- ☐ Make others happy
- ☐ Show love & support
- ☐ Challenge myself
- ☐ Feel good/have fun
- ☐ Complete overdue task
- ☐ Resolve something
- ☐ Make progress
- ☐ Relax

TUESDAY

"Wine [is] constant proof that God loves us and loves to see us happy."
—BENJAMIN FRANKLIN

DATE: __/__/__

One success I had today:

One redo I want:

One goal for tomorrow:

Why:

- ☐ Make others happy
- ☐ Show love & support
- ☐ Challenge myself
- ☐ Feel good/have fun
- ☐ Complete overdue task
- ☐ Resolve something
- ☐ Make progress
- ☐ Relax

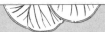

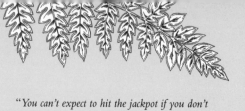

WEDNESDAY

DATE: __/__/__

"You can't expect to hit the jackpot if you don't put a few nickels in the machine."
—FLIP WILSON

One happiness today:

One screwup:

One intention for tomorrow:

Why:

- ☐ Make others happy
- ☐ Show love & support
- ☐ Challenge myself
- ☐ Feel good/have fun
- ☐ Complete overdue task
- ☐ Resolve something
- ☐ Make progress
- ☐ Relax

THURSDAY

DATE: __/__/__

"Knowing yourself is the beginning of all wisdom."
—ARISTOTLE

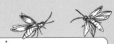

One success I had today:

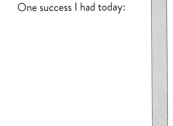

One redo I want:

One goal for tomorrow:

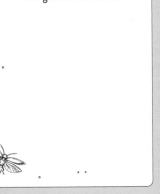

Why:

- ☐ Make others happy
- ☐ Show love & support
- ☐ Challenge myself
- ☐ Feel good/have fun
- ☐ Complete overdue task
- ☐ Resolve something
- ☐ Make progress
- ☐ Relax

"Never give up, for that is just the place and time that the tide will turn."
—HARRIET BEECHER STOWE

DATE: __/__/__

One happiness today:

One screwup:

One intention for tomorrow:

Why:

☐ Make others happy
☐ Show love & support
☐ Challenge myself
☐ Feel good/have fun
☐ Complete overdue task
☐ Resolve something
☐ Make progress
☐ Relax

"Write it on your heart that every day is the best day in the year." —**RALPH WALDO EMERSON**

WEEKEND

DATE: __/__/__

Success of the week:

Best experience of the week:

One treat planned for the weekend:

One inspiration/realization:

"There is nothing deep down inside us except what we have put there ourselves."
—RICHARD RORTY

One success I had today:

One redo I want:

One goal for tomorrow:

Why:

☐ Make others happy
☐ Show love & support
☐ Challenge myself
☐ Feel good/have fun
☐ Complete overdue task
☐ Resolve something
☐ Make progress
☐ Relax

"You can't wait for inspiration. You have to go after it with a club." —**JACK LONDON**

One happiness today:

One screwup:

One intention for tomorrow:

Why:

- ☐ Make others happy
- ☐ Show love & support
- ☐ Challenge myself
- ☐ Feel good/have fun
- ☐ Complete overdue task
- ☐ Resolve something
- ☐ Make progress
- ☐ Relax

DATE: __/__/__

"We may encounter many defeats, but we must not be defeated." —**MAYA ANGELOU**

One success I had today:

One redo I want:

One goal for tomorrow:

Why:

- ☐ Make others happy
- ☐ Show love & support
- ☐ Challenge myself
- ☐ Feel good/have fun
- ☐ Complete overdue task
- ☐ Resolve something
- ☐ Make progress
- ☐ Relax

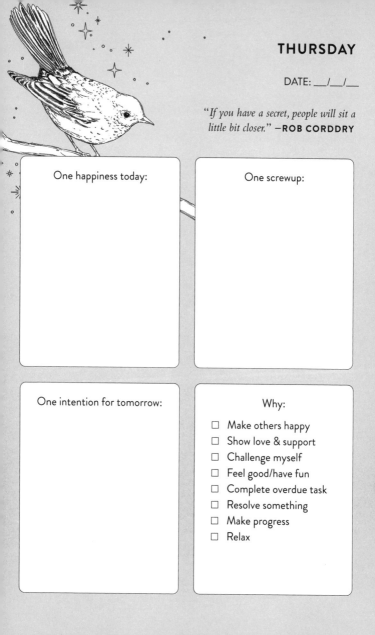

THURSDAY

DATE: __/__/__

"If you have a secret, people will sit a little bit closer." —**ROB CORDDRY**

One happiness today:

One screwup:

One intention for tomorrow:

Why:

- ☐ Make others happy
- ☐ Show love & support
- ☐ Challenge myself
- ☐ Feel good/have fun
- ☐ Complete overdue task
- ☐ Resolve something
- ☐ Make progress
- ☐ Relax

DATE: ___/___/___

"Your talent is God's gift to you. What you do with it is your gift back to God."
—LEO BUSCAGLIA

One success I had today:

One redo I want:

One goal for tomorrow:

Why:

- ☐ Make others happy
- ☐ Show love & support
- ☐ Challenge myself
- ☐ Feel good/have fun
- ☐ Complete overdue task
- ☐ Resolve something
- ☐ Make progress
- ☐ Relax

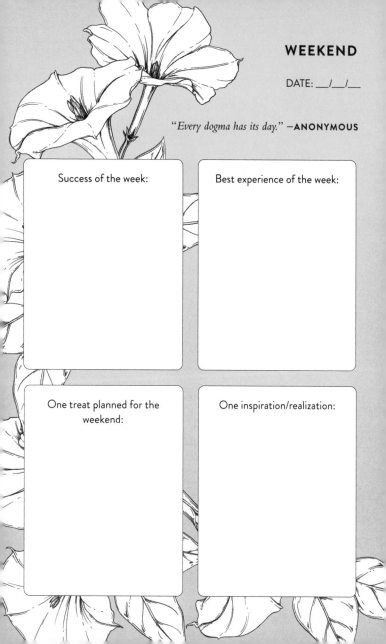

WEEKEND

DATE: __/__/__

"Every dogma has its day." —**ANONYMOUS**

Success of the week:

Best experience of the week:

One treat planned for the weekend:

One inspiration/realization:

MONDAY

DATE: __/__/__

"There's a way to do it better—find it."
—THOMAS A. EDISON

One happiness today:

One screwup:

One intention for tomorrow:

Why:

☐ Make others happy
☐ Show love & support
☐ Challenge myself
☐ Feel good/have fun
☐ Complete overdue task
☐ Resolve something
☐ Make progress
☐ Relax

*"No man is an island, entire of itself; every man is
a piece of the continent, a part of the main."*
–JOHN DONNE

DATE: __/__/__

One success I had today:

One redo I want:

One goal for tomorrow:

Why:

☐ Make others happy
☐ Show love & support
☐ Challenge myself
☐ Feel good/have fun
☐ Complete overdue task
☐ Resolve something
☐ Make progress
☐ Relax

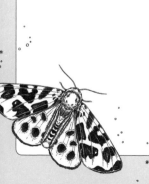

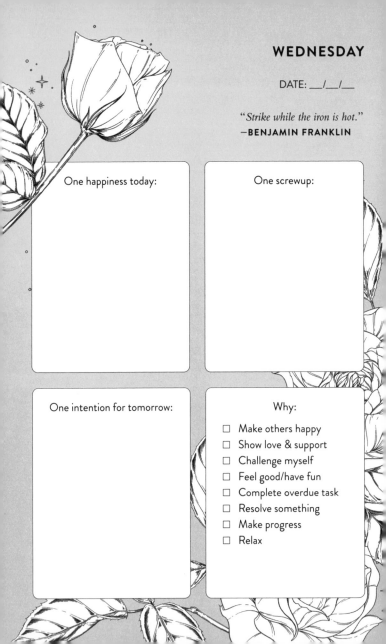

WEDNESDAY

DATE: __/__/__

"Strike while the iron is hot."
—**BENJAMIN FRANKLIN**

One happiness today:

One screwup:

One intention for tomorrow:

Why:

- ☐ Make others happy
- ☐ Show love & support
- ☐ Challenge myself
- ☐ Feel good/have fun
- ☐ Complete overdue task
- ☐ Resolve something
- ☐ Make progress
- ☐ Relax

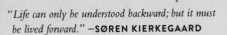

"Life can only be understood backward; but it must be lived forward." —**SØREN KIERKEGAARD**

DATE: __/__/__

One success I had today:

One redo I want:

Goal for tomorrow:

Why:

- ☐ Make others happy
- ☐ Show love & support
- ☐ Challenge myself
- ☐ Feel good/have fun
- ☐ Complete overdue task
- ☐ Resolve something
- ☐ Make progress
- ☐ Relax

"It is very important to know who you are. To make decisions. To show who you are."
—MALALA YOUSAFZAI

DATE: __/__/__

One happiness today:

One screwup:

One intention for tomorrow:

Why:

- ☐ Make others happy
- ☐ Show love & support
- ☐ Challenge myself
- ☐ Feel good/have fun
- ☐ Complete overdue task
- ☐ Resolve something
- ☐ Make progress
- ☐ Relax

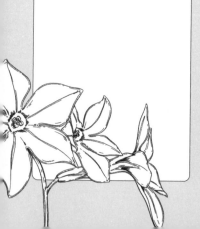

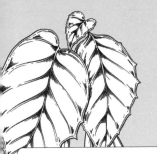

DATE: __/__/__

"Common sense is the collection of prejudices acquired by age eighteen."
—ALBERT EINSTEIN

Success of the week:

Best experience of the week:

One treat planned for the weekend:

One inspiration/realization:

DATE: __/__/__

"The key is to keep company only with people who uplift you, whose presence calls forth your best." —**EPICTETUS**

One success I had today:

One redo I want:

One goal for tomorrow:

Why:

- ☐ Make others happy
- ☐ Show love & support
- ☐ Challenge myself
- ☐ Feel good/have fun
- ☐ Complete overdue task
- ☐ Resolve something
- ☐ Make progress
- ☐ Relax

TUESDAY

DATE: ___/___/___

"With freedom, books, flowers, and the moon, who could not be perfectly happy?"
—OSCAR WILDE

One happiness today:

One screwup:

One intention for tomorrow:

Why:

- ☐ Make others happy
- ☐ Show love & support
- ☐ Challenge myself
- ☐ Feel good/have fun
- ☐ Complete overdue task
- ☐ Resolve something
- ☐ Make progress
- ☐ Relax

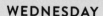

DATE: __/__/__

"You can't cross the sea merely by standing and staring at the water."
—RABINDRANATH TAGORE

One success I had today:

One redo I want:

One goal for tomorrow:

Why:

- ☐ Make others happy
- ☐ Show love & support
- ☐ Challenge myself
- ☐ Feel good/have fun
- ☐ Complete overdue task
- ☐ Resolve something
- ☐ Make progress
- ☐ Relax

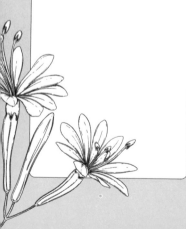

DATE: ___/___/___

"If at first you don't succeed, blame your parents."
—MARCELENE COX

One happiness today:

One screwup:

One intention for tomorrow:

Why:

- ☐ Make others happy
- ☐ Show love & support
- ☐ Challenge myself
- ☐ Feel good/have fun
- ☐ Complete overdue task
- ☐ Resolve something
- ☐ Make progress
- ☐ Relax

DATE: __/__/__

"I believe one of the greatest pleasures of life is to curl up one's legs in bed." **—LIN YUTANG**

One success I had today:

One redo I want:

One goal for tomorrow:

Why:

☐ Make others happy
☐ Show love & support
☐ Challenge myself
☐ Feel good/have fun
☐ Complete overdue task
☐ Resolve something
☐ Make progress
☐ Relax

"Life is going to give you just what you put in it. Put your whole heart in everything you do, and pray, then you can wait." —**MAYA ANGELOU**

Success of the week:

Best experience of the week:

One treat planned for the weekend:

One inspiration/realization:

"We make the world we live in and shape our own environment." —**ORISON SWETT MARDEN**

DATE: __/__/__

One happiness today:

One screwup:

One intention for tomorrow:

Why:

- [ ] Make others happy
- [ ] Show love & support
- [ ] Challenge myself
- [ ] Feel good/have fun
- [ ] Complete overdue task
- [ ] Resolve something
- [ ] Make progress
- [ ] Relax

"Laugh as much as you choose, but you will not laugh me out of my opinion." —**JANE AUSTEN**

DATE: __/__/__

One success I had today:

One redo I want:

One goal for tomorrow:

Why:

- [ ] Make others happy
- [ ] Show love & support
- [ ] Challenge myself
- [ ] Feel good/have fun
- [ ] Complete overdue task
- [ ] Resolve something
- [ ] Make progress
- [ ] Relax

"Never, never, never give up."
—WINSTON CHURCHILL

DATE: __/__/__

One happiness today:

One screwup:

One intention for tomorrow:

Why:

- ☐ Make others happy
- ☐ Show love & support
- ☐ Challenge myself
- ☐ Feel good/have fun
- ☐ Complete overdue task
- ☐ Resolve something
- ☐ Make progress
- ☐ Relax

THURSDAY

"Set yourself earnestly to see what you are made to do, and then set yourself earnestly to do it."
—PHILLIPS BROOKS

One success I had today:

One redo I want:

One goal for tomorrow:

Why:

☐ Make others happy
☐ Show love & support
☐ Challenge myself
☐ Feel good/have fun
☐ Complete overdue task
☐ Resolve something
☐ Make progress
☐ Relax

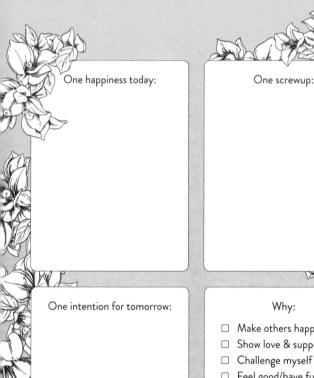

"If you want to conquer fear, don't sit home and think about it. Go out and get busy."
—DALE CARNEGIE

FRIDAY

DATE: __/__/__

One happiness today:

One screwup:

One intention for tomorrow:

Why:

☐ Make others happy
☐ Show love & support
☐ Challenge myself
☐ Feel good/have fun
☐ Complete overdue task
☐ Resolve something
☐ Make progress
☐ Relax

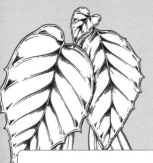

WEEKEND

DATE: __/__/__

"I'm looking for a blessing not in disguise."
—JEROME K. JEROME

Success of the week:

Best experience of the week:

One treat planned for the weekend:

One inspiration/realization:

"If you ask me what I came into this life to do, I, an artist, will answer you: I came to live out loud."
—EMILE ZOLA

DATE: ___/___/___

One success I had today:

One redo I want:

One goal for tomorrow:

Why:

- ☐ Make others happy
- ☐ Show love & support
- ☐ Challenge myself
- ☐ Feel good/have fun
- ☐ Complete overdue task
- ☐ Resolve something
- ☐ Make progress
- ☐ Relax

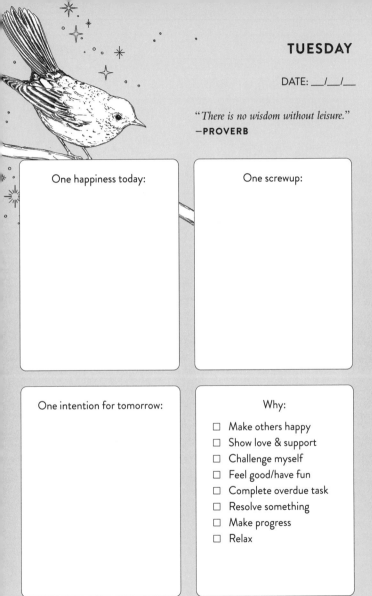

TUESDAY

DATE: __/__/__

"There is no wisdom without leisure."
—PROVERB

One happiness today:

One screwup:

One intention for tomorrow:

Why:

- ☐ Make others happy
- ☐ Show love & support
- ☐ Challenge myself
- ☐ Feel good/have fun
- ☐ Complete overdue task
- ☐ Resolve something
- ☐ Make progress
- ☐ Relax

WEDNESDAY

"Press forward. Do not stop, do not linger in your journey, but strive for the mark set before you."
—GEORGE WHITEFIELD

DATE: __/__/__

One success I had today:

One redo I want:

One goal for tomorrow:

Why:

- ☐ Make others happy
- ☐ Show love & support
- ☐ Challenge myself
- ☐ Feel good/have fun
- ☐ Complete overdue task
- ☐ Resolve something
- ☐ Make progress
- ☐ Relax

DATE: __/__/__

"The world is all gates, all opportunities, strings of tension waiting to be struck."
—RALPH WALDO EMERSON

One happiness today:

One screwup:

One intention for tomorrow:

Why:

☐ Make others happy
☐ Show love & support
☐ Challenge myself
☐ Feel good/have fun
☐ Complete overdue task
☐ Resolve something
☐ Make progress
☐ Relax

FRIDAY

DATE: ___/___/___

"It's always too early to quit."
—NORMAN VINCENT PEALE

One success I had today:

One redo I want:

One goal for tomorrow:

Why:

- ☐ Make others happy
- ☐ Show love & support
- ☐ Challenge myself
- ☐ Feel good/have fun
- ☐ Complete overdue task
- ☐ Resolve something
- ☐ Make progress
- ☐ Relax

"I will be calm. I will be mistress of myself."
—JANE AUSTEN

DATE: ___/___/___

Success of the week:

Best experience of the week:

One treat planned for the weekend:

One inspiration/realization:

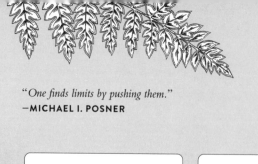

DATE: __/__/__

"One finds limits by pushing them."
—MICHAEL I. POSNER

One happiness today:

One screwup:

One intention for tomorrow:

Why:

- ☐ Make others happy
- ☐ Show love & support
- ☐ Challenge myself
- ☐ Feel good/have fun
- ☐ Complete overdue task
- ☐ Resolve something
- ☐ Make progress
- ☐ Relax

"Whether I come to my own to-day or in ten thousand or ten million years, I can cheerfully take it now, or with equal cheerfulness I can wait."
—WALT WHITMAN

One success I had today:

One redo I want:

One goal for tomorrow:

Why:
- [ ] Make others happy
- [ ] Show love & support
- [ ] Challenge myself
- [ ] Feel good/have fun
- [ ] Complete overdue task
- [ ] Resolve something
- [ ] Make progress
- [ ] Relax

"You can't build a reputation on what you're going to do." —**HENRY FORD**

DATE: __/__/__

One happiness today:

One screwup:

One intention for tomorrow:

Why:

- ☐ Make others happy
- ☐ Show love & support
- ☐ Challenge myself
- ☐ Feel good/have fun
- ☐ Complete overdue task
- ☐ Resolve something
- ☐ Make progress
- ☐ Relax

THURSDAY

"We owe a lot to Thomas Edison—if it wasn't for him, we'd be watching TV by candlelight."
—MILTON BERLE

DATE: __/__/__

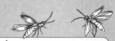

One success I had today:

One redo I want:

One goal for tomorrow:

Why:

☐ Make others happy
☐ Show love & support
☐ Challenge myself
☐ Feel good/have fun
☐ Complete overdue task
☐ Resolve something
☐ Make progress
☐ Relax

"You create your opportunities by asking for them."
—SHAKTI GAWAIN

DATE: __/__/__

One happiness today:

One screwup:

One intention for tomorrow:

Why:

- ☐ Make others happy
- ☐ Show love & support
- ☐ Challenge myself
- ☐ Feel good/have fun
- ☐ Complete overdue task
- ☐ Resolve something
- ☐ Make progress
- ☐ Relax

"Have patience with everything that remains unsolved in your heart."
—RAINER MARIA RILKE

DATE: __/__/__

Success of the week:

Best experience of the week:

One treat planned for the weekend:

One inspiration/realization:

"Deserve your dream." —OCTAVIO PAZ

One happiness today:

One screwup:

One intention for tomorrow:

Why:

☐ Make others happy
☐ Show love & support
☐ Challenge myself
☐ Feel good/have fun
☐ Complete overdue task
☐ Resolve something
☐ Make progress
☐ Relax

DATE: __/__/__

"Every man has his follies—and often they are the most interesting thing he has got."
—JOSH BILLINGS

One success I had today:

One redo I want:

One goal for tomorrow:

Why:

☐ Make others happy
☐ Show love & support
☐ Challenge myself
☐ Feel good/have fun
☐ Complete overdue task
☐ Resolve something
☐ Make progress
☐ Relax

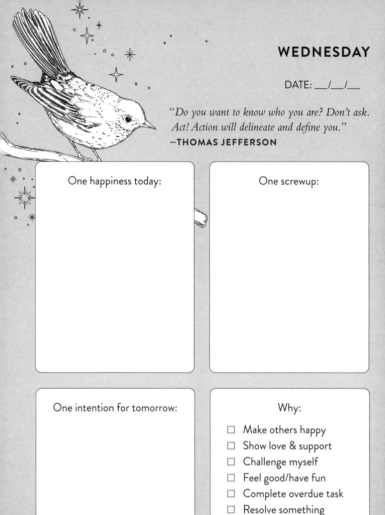

WEDNESDAY

DATE: __/__/__

"Do you want to know who you are? Don't ask. Act! Action will delineate and define you."
—THOMAS JEFFERSON

One happiness today:

One screwup:

One intention for tomorrow:

Why:

- ☐ Make others happy
- ☐ Show love & support
- ☐ Challenge myself
- ☐ Feel good/have fun
- ☐ Complete overdue task
- ☐ Resolve something
- ☐ Make progress
- ☐ Relax

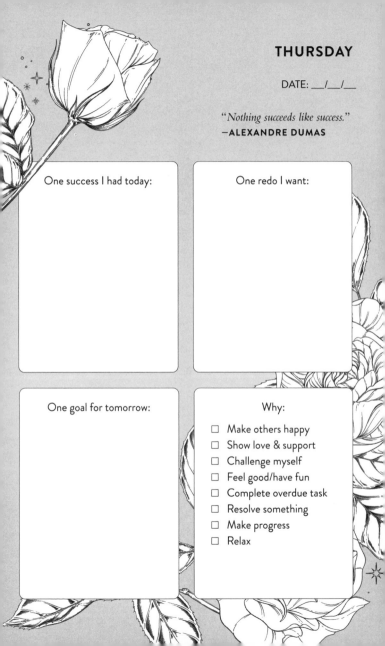

THURSDAY

DATE: __/__/__

"Nothing succeeds like success."
—ALEXANDRE DUMAS

One success I had today:

One redo I want:

One goal for tomorrow:

Why:

- ☐ Make others happy
- ☐ Show love & support
- ☐ Challenge myself
- ☐ Feel good/have fun
- ☐ Complete overdue task
- ☐ Resolve something
- ☐ Make progress
- ☐ Relax

DATE: __/__/__

"The more we do, the more we can do."
—WILLIAM HAZLITT

One happiness today:

One screwup:

One intention for tomorrow:

Why:

- ☐ Make others happy
- ☐ Show love & support
- ☐ Challenge myself
- ☐ Feel good/have fun
- ☐ Complete overdue task
- ☐ Resolve something
- ☐ Make progress
- ☐ Relax

"We may not be able to make all our dreams come true, but it is an astonishing thing how often . . . we can 'dream true.'" —**ELEANOR ROOSEVELT**

Success of the week:

Best experience of the week:

One treat planned for the weekend:

One inspiration/realization:

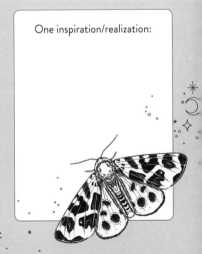

"We should not give up and we should not allow the problem to defeat us."
—A. P. J. ABDUL KALAM

DATE: __/__/__

One success I had today:

One redo I want:

One goal for tomorrow:

Why:

☐ Make others happy
☐ Show love & support
☐ Challenge myself
☐ Feel good/have fun
☐ Complete overdue task
☐ Resolve something
☐ Make progress
☐ Relax

"A world full of happiness is not beyond human power to create." —**BERTRAND RUSSELL**

DATE: ___/___/___

One happiness today:

One screwup:

One intention for tomorrow:

Why:

- ☐ Make others happy
- ☐ Show love & support
- ☐ Challenge myself
- ☐ Feel good/have fun
- ☐ Complete overdue task
- ☐ Resolve something
- ☐ Make progress
- ☐ Relax

"I think people who are creative are the luckiest people on earth. . . . Do what you love and you will find the way to get it out to the world."
—JUDY GARLAND

WEDNESDAY

DATE: __/__/__

One success I had today:

One redo I want:

One goal for tomorrow:

Why:

- ☐ Make others happy
- ☐ Show love & support
- ☐ Challenge myself
- ☐ Feel good/have fun
- ☐ Complete overdue task
- ☐ Resolve something
- ☐ Make progress
- ☐ Relax

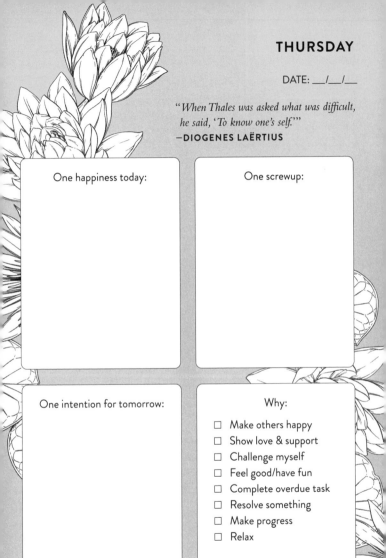

THURSDAY

DATE: ___/___/___

"When Thales was asked what was difficult, he said, 'To know one's self.'"
—DIOGENES LAËRTIUS

One happiness today:

One screwup:

One intention for tomorrow:

Why:

- ☐ Make others happy
- ☐ Show love & support
- ☐ Challenge myself
- ☐ Feel good/have fun
- ☐ Complete overdue task
- ☐ Resolve something
- ☐ Make progress
- ☐ Relax

FRIDAY

"Wherever you are—be all there." **–JIM ELLIOT**

DATE: __/__/__

One success I had today:

One redo I want:

One goal for tomorrow:

Why:

- ☐ Make others happy
- ☐ Show love & support
- ☐ Challenge myself
- ☐ Feel good/have fun
- ☐ Complete overdue task
- ☐ Resolve something
- ☐ Make progress
- ☐ Relax

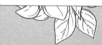

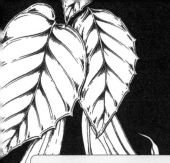

A TIME TO REVIEW

DATE: __/__/__

What has changed for me?

What themes recurred over the year?

What do I now want to change?

Why:

- [ ] It was not serving me well
- [ ] It is not my business
- [ ] To grow stronger
- [ ] To be more loving
- [ ] To be more resilient
- [ ] To be more determined

DATE: ___/___/___

*"I know where I'm going and I know the truth,
and I don't have to be what you want me to be.
I'm free to be what I want."*
—MUHAMMAD ALI

One happiness today:

One screwup:

One intention for tomorrow:

Why:

- ☐ Make others happy
- ☐ Show love & support
- ☐ Challenge myself
- ☐ Feel good/have fun
- ☐ Complete overdue task
- ☐ Resolve something
- ☐ Make progress
- ☐ Relax

"Dreams, books, are each a world."
—WILLIAM WORDSWORTH

DATE: __/__/__

One success I had today:

One redo I want:

One goal for tomorrow:

Why:

- ☐ Make others happy
- ☐ Show love & support
- ☐ Challenge myself
- ☐ Feel good/have fun
- ☐ Complete overdue task
- ☐ Resolve something
- ☐ Make progress
- ☐ Relax

"After a storm comes a calm."
—PROVERB

DATE: __/__/__

One happiness today:

One screwup:

One intention for tomorrow:

Why:

- ☐ Make others happy
- ☐ Show love & support
- ☐ Challenge myself
- ☐ Feel good/have fun
- ☐ Complete overdue task
- ☐ Resolve something
- ☐ Make progress
- ☐ Relax

DATE: __/__/__

"Lead us not into temptation. Just tell us where it is; we'll find it." **—SAM LEVENSON**

One success I had today:

One redo I want:

One goal for tomorrow:

Why:

☐ Make others happy
☐ Show love & support
☐ Challenge myself
☐ Feel good/have fun
☐ Complete overdue task
☐ Resolve something
☐ Make progress
☐ Relax

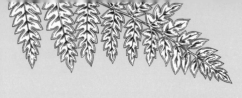

"If you don't like how things are, change it! You're not a tree." —**JIM ROHN**

One happiness today:

One screwup:

One intention for tomorrow:

Why:

- ☐ Make others happy
- ☐ Show love & support
- ☐ Challenge myself
- ☐ Feel good/have fun
- ☐ Complete overdue task
- ☐ Resolve something
- ☐ Make progress
- ☐ Relax

DATE: __/__/__

"Beauty is everywhere, and beauty is only two fingers'-breadth from goodness."
—VIRGINIA WOOLF

Success of the week:

Best experience of the week:

One treat planned for the weekend:

One inspiration/realization:

MONDAY

DATE: ___/___/___

"Only rarely can we repay those people who helped us, but we can pass that help along to others."
—LUCILLE BALL

One success I had today:

One redo I want:

One goal for tomorrow:

Why:
- ☐ Make others happy
- ☐ Show love & support
- ☐ Challenge myself
- ☐ Feel good/have fun
- ☐ Complete overdue task
- ☐ Resolve something
- ☐ Make progress
- ☐ Relax

TUESDAY

"None of my inventions came by accident. I see a worthwhile need to be met and I make trial after trial until it comes." **–THOMAS A. EDISON**

DATE: __/__/__

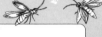

One happiness today:

One screwup:

One intention for tomorrow:

Why:

☐ Make others happy
☐ Show love & support
☐ Challenge myself
☐ Feel good/have fun
☐ Complete overdue task
☐ Resolve something
☐ Make progress
☐ Relax

DATE: __/__/__

"A somebody was once a nobody who wanted to and did." **–JAMES BURROUGHS**

One success I had today:

One redo I want:

One goal for tomorrow:

Why:

- ☐ Make others happy
- ☐ Show love & support
- ☐ Challenge myself
- ☐ Feel good/have fun
- ☐ Complete overdue task
- ☐ Resolve something
- ☐ Make progress
- ☐ Relax

"Mend when thou canst; be better at thy leisure."
—WILLIAM SHAKESPEARE

DATE: ___/___/___

One happiness today:

One screwup:

One intention for tomorrow:

Why:

☐ Make others happy
☐ Show love & support
☐ Challenge myself
☐ Feel good/have fun
☐ Complete overdue task
☐ Resolve something
☐ Make progress
☐ Relax

"It's a good thing to turn your mind upside down now and then, like an hourglass, to let the particles run the other way."
—CHRISTOPHER MORLEY

FRIDAY

DATE: __/__/__

One success I had today:

One redo I want:

One goal for tomorrow:

Why:

- ☐ Make others happy
- ☐ Show love & support
- ☐ Challenge myself
- ☐ Feel good/have fun
- ☐ Complete overdue task
- ☐ Resolve something
- ☐ Make progress
- ☐ Relax

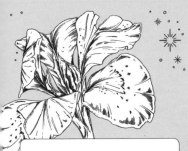

"Macho does not prove mucho."
—ZSA ZSA GABOR

Success of the week:

Best experience of the week:

One treat planned for the weekend:

One inspiration/realization:

MONDAY

DATE: __/__/__

"A goal is a dream with a deadline."
—NAPOLEON HILL

One happiness today:

One screwup:

One intention for tomorrow:

Why:

- ☐ Make others happy
- ☐ Show love & support
- ☐ Challenge myself
- ☐ Feel good/have fun
- ☐ Complete overdue task
- ☐ Resolve something
- ☐ Make progress
- ☐ Relax

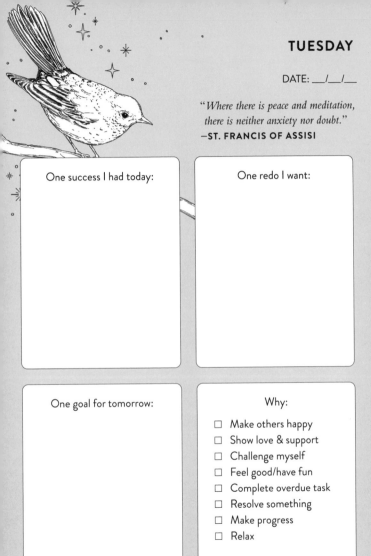

TUESDAY

DATE: __/__/__

"Where there is peace and meditation, there is neither anxiety nor doubt."
—ST. FRANCIS OF ASSISI

One success I had today:

One redo I want:

One goal for tomorrow:

Why:

- ☐ Make others happy
- ☐ Show love & support
- ☐ Challenge myself
- ☐ Feel good/have fun
- ☐ Complete overdue task
- ☐ Resolve something
- ☐ Make progress
- ☐ Relax

WEDNESDAY

DATE: __/__/__

"We aim above the mark to hit the mark."
—RALPH WALDO EMERSON

One happiness today:

One screwup:

One intention for tomorrow:

Why:

- ☐ Make others happy
- ☐ Show love & support
- ☐ Challenge myself
- ☐ Feel good/have fun
- ☐ Complete overdue task
- ☐ Resolve something
- ☐ Make progress
- ☐ Relax

THURSDAY

DATE: __/__/__

"There are lots of people who mistake their imagination for their memory."
—JOSH BILLINGS

One success I had today:

One redo I want:

One goal for tomorrow:

Why:

- [ ] Make others happy
- [ ] Show love & support
- [ ] Challenge myself
- [ ] Feel good/have fun
- [ ] Complete overdue task
- [ ] Resolve something
- [ ] Make progress
- [ ] Relax

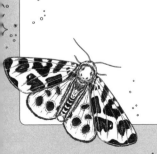

"Do your work with your whole heart, and you will succeed—there's so little competition."
—ELBERT HUBBARD

DATE: __/__/__

One happiness today:

One screwup:

One intention for tomorrow:

Why:

- ☐ Make others happy
- ☐ Show love & support
- ☐ Challenge myself
- ☐ Feel good/have fun
- ☐ Complete overdue task
- ☐ Resolve something
- ☐ Make progress
- ☐ Relax

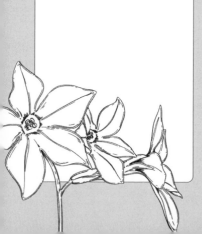

"One of the disadvantages of wine is that it makes a man mistake words for thoughts."
—SAMUEL JOHNSON

Success of the week:

Best experience of the week:

One treat planned for the weekend:

One inspiration/realization:

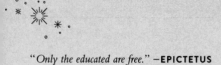

"*Only the educated are free.*" **—EPICTETUS**

DATE: ___/___/___

One success I had today:

One redo I want:

One goal for tomorrow:

Why:

- ☐ Make others happy
- ☐ Show love & support
- ☐ Challenge myself
- ☐ Feel good/have fun
- ☐ Complete overdue task
- ☐ Resolve something
- ☐ Make progress
- ☐ Relax

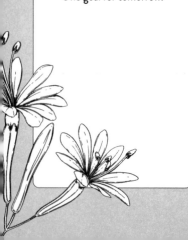

DATE: __/__/__

"To travel hopefully is a better thing than to arrive." —**ROBERT LOUIS STEVENSON**

One happiness today:

One screwup:

One intention for tomorrow:

Why:

- ☐ Make others happy
- ☐ Show love & support
- ☐ Challenge myself
- ☐ Feel good/have fun
- ☐ Complete overdue task
- ☐ Resolve something
- ☐ Make progress
- ☐ Relax

WEDNESDAY

"Do something wonderful, people may imitate it."
—ALBERT SCHWEITZER

DATE: __/__/__

One success I had today:

One redo I want:

One goal for tomorrow:

Why:

- ☐ Make others happy
- ☐ Show love & support
- ☐ Challenge myself
- ☐ Feel good/have fun
- ☐ Complete overdue task
- ☐ Resolve something
- ☐ Make progress
- ☐ Relax

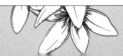

THURSDAY

DATE: __/__/__

"Be gentle to all and stern with yourself."
—SAINT THERESA OF ÁVILA

One happiness today:

One screwup:

One intention for tomorrow:

Why:

☐ Make others happy
☐ Show love & support
☐ Challenge myself
☐ Feel good/have fun
☐ Complete overdue task
☐ Resolve something
☐ Make progress
☐ Relax

"Hitch your wagon to a star."
—RALPH WALDO EMERSON

DATE: __/__/__

One success I had today:

One redo I want:

One goal for tomorrow:

Why:

- ☐ Make others happy
- ☐ Show love & support
- ☐ Challenge myself
- ☐ Feel good/have fun
- ☐ Complete overdue task
- ☐ Resolve something
- ☐ Make progress
- ☐ Relax

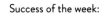

"Knowing others is wisdom; knowing yourself is enlightenment." **—LAO TZU**

DATE: __/__/__

Success of the week:

Best experience of the week:

One treat planned for the weekend:

One inspiration/realization:

MONDAY

DATE: __/__/__

"To be a good loser is to learn how to win."
—CARL SANDBURG

One happiness today:

One screwup:

One intention for tomorrow:

Why:

- ☐ Make others happy
- ☐ Show love & support
- ☐ Challenge myself
- ☐ Feel good/have fun
- ☐ Complete overdue task
- ☐ Resolve something
- ☐ Make progress
- ☐ Relax

"To accomplish great things we must not only act, but also dream; not only plan, but also believe."
—ANATOLE FRANCE

One success I had today:

One redo I want:

One goal for tomorrow:

Why:

- [ ] Make others happy
- [ ] Show love & support
- [ ] Challenge myself
- [ ] Feel good/have fun
- [ ] Complete overdue task
- [ ] Resolve something
- [ ] Make progress
- [ ] Relax

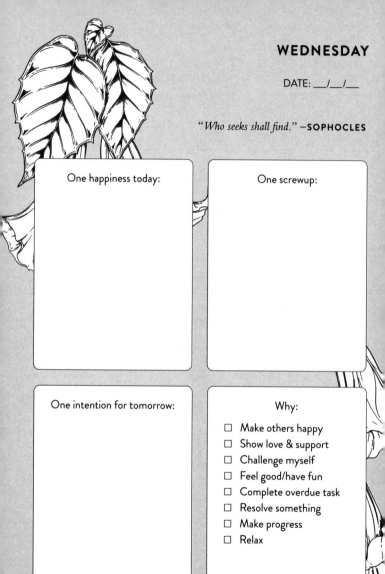

WEDNESDAY

DATE: __/__/__

"Who seeks shall find." —**SOPHOCLES**

One happiness today:

One screwup:

One intention for tomorrow:

Why:

- ☐ Make others happy
- ☐ Show love & support
- ☐ Challenge myself
- ☐ Feel good/have fun
- ☐ Complete overdue task
- ☐ Resolve something
- ☐ Make progress
- ☐ Relax

THURSDAY

DATE: __/__/__

One success I had today:

One redo I want:

One goal for tomorrow:

Why:

- ☐ Make others happy
- ☐ Show love & support
- ☐ Challenge myself
- ☐ Feel good/have fun
- ☐ Complete overdue task
- ☐ Resolve something
- ☐ Make progress
- ☐ Relax

*"Start with a clean slate and spend all your
energies in keeping it clean for the future."*
—ORISON SWETT MARDEN

DATE: __/__/__

One happiness today:

One screwup:

One intention for tomorrow:

Why:

- ☐ Make others happy
- ☐ Show love & support
- ☐ Challenge myself
- ☐ Feel good/have fun
- ☐ Complete overdue task
- ☐ Resolve something
- ☐ Make progress
- ☐ Relax

WEEKEND

DATE: __/__/__

*"Go into your own ground and learn to know
yourself there."* —**MEISTER ECKHART**

Success of the week:

Best experience of the week:

One treat planned for the
weekend:

One inspiration/realization:

DATE: __/__/__

One success I had today:

One redo I want:

One goal for tomorrow:

Why:

- ☐ Make others happy
- ☐ Show love & support
- ☐ Challenge myself
- ☐ Feel good/have fun
- ☐ Complete overdue task
- ☐ Resolve something
- ☐ Make progress
- ☐ Relax

TUESDAY

*"Have enough sense to know, ahead of time, when
your skills will not extend to wallpapering."*
—MARILYN VOS SAVANT

DATE: __/__/__

One happiness today:

One screwup:

One intention for tomorrow:

Why:

- ☐ Make others happy
- ☐ Show love & support
- ☐ Challenge myself
- ☐ Feel good/have fun
- ☐ Complete overdue task
- ☐ Resolve something
- ☐ Make progress
- ☐ Relax

"The past cannot be changed. The future is yet in your power." —**ANONYMOUS**

DATE: __/__/__

One success I had today:

One redo I want:

One goal for tomorrow:

Why:

- ☐ Make others happy
- ☐ Show love & support
- ☐ Challenge myself
- ☐ Feel good/have fun
- ☐ Complete overdue task
- ☐ Resolve something
- ☐ Make progress
- ☐ Relax

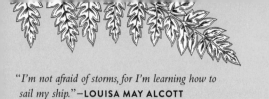

"I'm not afraid of storms, for I'm learning how to sail my ship." —**LOUISA MAY ALCOTT**

DATE: ___/___/___

One happiness today:

One screwup:

One intention for tomorrow:

Why:

- ☐ Make others happy
- ☐ Show love & support
- ☐ Challenge myself
- ☐ Feel good/have fun
- ☐ Complete overdue task
- ☐ Resolve something
- ☐ Make progress
- ☐ Relax

"Pursue one great decisive aim with force and determination." —**CARL VON CLAUSEWITZ**

DATE: __/__/__

One success I had today:

One redo I want:

One goal for tomorrow:

Why:

- ☐ Make others happy
- ☐ Show love & support
- ☐ Challenge myself
- ☐ Feel good/have fun
- ☐ Complete overdue task
- ☐ Resolve something
- ☐ Make progress
- ☐ Relax

WEEKEND

"Happiness is inward, and not outward; and so, it does not depend on what we have, but on what we are." —**HENRY VAN DYKE**

DATE: __/__/__

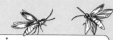

Success of the week:

Best experience of the week:

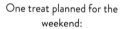

One treat planned for the weekend:

One inspiration/realization:

"I was motivated to be different in part because I was different." —**DONNA BRAZILE**

DATE: __/__/__

One happiness today:

One screwup:

One intention for tomorrow:

Why:

- ☐ Make others happy
- ☐ Show love & support
- ☐ Challenge myself
- ☐ Feel good/have fun
- ☐ Complete overdue task
- ☐ Resolve something
- ☐ Make progress
- ☐ Relax

TUESDAY

"Gratitude is a divine emotion. It fills the heart, but not to bursting; it warms it, but not to fever."
—CHARLOTTE BRONTË

DATE: __/__/__

One success I had today:

One redo I want:

One goal for tomorrow:

Why:

- ☐ Make others happy
- ☐ Show love & support
- ☐ Challenge myself
- ☐ Feel good/have fun
- ☐ Complete overdue task
- ☐ Resolve something
- ☐ Make progress
- ☐ Relax

WEDNESDAY

DATE: __/__/__

"Don't give up. Don't lose hope. Don't sell out." —**CHRISTOPHER REEVE**

One happiness today:

One screwup:

One intention for tomorrow:

Why:

- ☐ Make others happy
- ☐ Show love & support
- ☐ Challenge myself
- ☐ Feel good/have fun
- ☐ Complete overdue task
- ☐ Resolve something
- ☐ Make progress
- ☐ Relax

THURSDAY

DATE: __/__/__

"Memory . . . is the diary that we all carry about with us." **—OSCAR WILDE**

One success I had today:

One redo I want:

One goal for tomorrow:

Why:

- ☐ Make others happy
- ☐ Show love & support
- ☐ Challenge myself
- ☐ Feel good/have fun
- ☐ Complete overdue task
- ☐ Resolve something
- ☐ Make progress
- ☐ Relax

FRIDAY

DATE: __/__/__

"Know or listen to those who know."
—BALTASAR GRACIÁN

One happiness today:

One screwup:

One intention for tomorrow:

Why:

- ☐ Make others happy
- ☐ Show love & support
- ☐ Challenge myself
- ☐ Feel good/have fun
- ☐ Complete overdue task
- ☐ Resolve something
- ☐ Make progress
- ☐ Relax

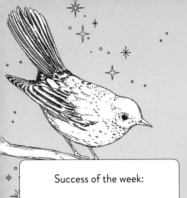

WEEKEND

DATE: __/__/__

"A nickel ain't worth a dime anymore."
—YOGI BERRA

Success of the week:

Best experience of the week:

One treat planned for the weekend:

One inspiration/realization:

MONDAY

DATE: __/__/__

"You have to make it happen."
—DENIS DIDEROT

One happiness today:

One screwup:

One intention for tomorrow:

Why:

- ☐ Make others happy
- ☐ Show love & support
- ☐ Challenge myself
- ☐ Feel good/have fun
- ☐ Complete overdue task
- ☐ Resolve something
- ☐ Make progress
- ☐ Relax

"A pessimist is a person who has had to listen to too many optimists." **–DON MARQUIS**

DATE: __/__/__

One success I had today:

One redo I want:

One goal for tomorrow:

Why:

- ☐ Make others happy
- ☐ Show love & support
- ☐ Challenge myself
- ☐ Feel good/have fun
- ☐ Complete overdue task
- ☐ Resolve something
- ☐ Make progress
- ☐ Relax

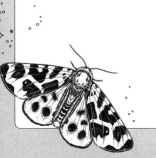

"The wise does at once what the fool does at last."
—BALTASAR GRACIÁN

DATE: ___/___/___

One happiness today:

One screwup:

One intention for tomorrow:

Why:

- ☐ Make others happy
- ☐ Show love & support
- ☐ Challenge myself
- ☐ Feel good/have fun
- ☐ Complete overdue task
- ☐ Resolve something
- ☐ Make progress
- ☐ Relax

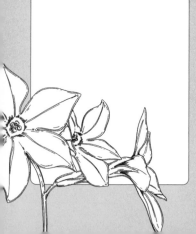

DATE: __/__/__

"Knowing others is wisdom; knowing yourself is enlightenment." **—LAO TZU**

One success I had today:

One redo I want:

One goal for tomorrow:

Why:

- ☐ Make others happy
- ☐ Show love & support
- ☐ Challenge myself
- ☐ Feel good/have fun
- ☐ Complete overdue task
- ☐ Resolve something
- ☐ Make progress
- ☐ Relax

DATE: __/__/__

"I know not age, nor weariness, nor defeat."
—ROSE KENNEDY

One happiness today:

One screwup:

One intention for tomorrow:

Why:

- ☐ Make others happy
- ☐ Show love & support
- ☐ Challenge myself
- ☐ Feel good/have fun
- ☐ Complete overdue task
- ☐ Resolve something
- ☐ Make progress
- ☐ Relax

WEEKEND

DATE: __/__/__

"Oh bed! oh bed! delicious bed! That heaven upon earth to the weary head." **—THOMAS HOOD**

Success of the week:

Best experience of the week:

One treat planned for the weekend:

One inspiration/realization:

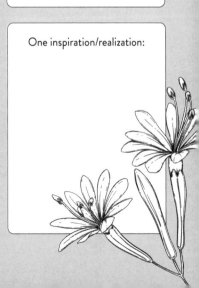

DATE: __/__/__

"Begin to be now what you will be hereafter."
—WILLIAM JAMES

One success I had today:

One redo I want:

One goal for tomorrow:

Why:

- ☐ Make others happy
- ☐ Show love & support
- ☐ Challenge myself
- ☐ Feel good/have fun
- ☐ Complete overdue task
- ☐ Resolve something
- ☐ Make progress
- ☐ Relax

"You can't use up creativity. The more you use, the more you have." —**MAYA ANGELOU**

DATE: __/__/__

One happiness today:

One screwup:

One intention for tomorrow:

Why:

- ☐ Make others happy
- ☐ Show love & support
- ☐ Challenge myself
- ☐ Feel good/have fun
- ☐ Complete overdue task
- ☐ Resolve something
- ☐ Make progress
- ☐ Relax

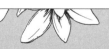

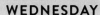

DATE: __/__/__

"March on. Do not tarry. To go forward is to move toward perfection. March on and fear not the thorns or the sharp stones on life's path."
—KHALIL GIBRAN

One success I had today:

One redo I want:

One goal for tomorrow:

Why:

- ☐ Make others happy
- ☐ Show love & support
- ☐ Challenge myself
- ☐ Feel good/have fun
- ☐ Complete overdue task
- ☐ Resolve something
- ☐ Make progress
- ☐ Relax

DATE: __/__/__

"Memories are like mulligatawny soup in a cheap restaurant. It is best not to stir them."
—P. G. WODEHOUSE

One happiness today:

One screwup:

One intention for tomorrow:

Why:

☐ Make others happy
☐ Show love & support
☐ Challenge myself
☐ Feel good/have fun
☐ Complete overdue task
☐ Resolve something
☐ Make progress
☐ Relax

"True happiness involves the full use of one's power and talents." **—JOHN W. GARDNER**

DATE: __/__/__

One success I had today:

One redo I want:

One goal for tomorrow:

Why:

- ☐ Make others happy
- ☐ Show love & support
- ☐ Challenge myself
- ☐ Feel good/have fun
- ☐ Complete overdue task
- ☐ Resolve something
- ☐ Make progress
- ☐ Relax

"We should remember that just as a positive outlook on life can promote good health, so can everyday acts of kindness." —**HILLARY CLINTON**

Success of the week:

Best experience of the week:

One treat planned for the weekend:

One inspiration/realization:

"One may miss the mark by aiming too high as too low." —**THOMAS FULLER**

DATE: __/__/__

One happiness today:

One screwup:

One intention for tomorrow:

Why:

- ☐ Make others happy
- ☐ Show love & support
- ☐ Challenge myself
- ☐ Feel good/have fun
- ☐ Complete overdue task
- ☐ Resolve something
- ☐ Make progress
- ☐ Relax

TUESDAY

DATE: __/__/__

"Unconsciously our characters shape themselves to meet the requirements which our dreams put upon our life." —**ELEANOR ROOSEVELT**

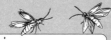

One success I had today:

One redo I want:

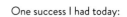

One goal for tomorrow:

Why:

- ☐ Make others happy
- ☐ Show love & support
- ☐ Challenge myself
- ☐ Feel good/have fun
- ☐ Complete overdue task
- ☐ Resolve something
- ☐ Make progress
- ☐ Relax

WEDNESDAY

"What can be explained is not poetry."
—JOHN BUTLER YEATS

DATE: __/__/__

One happiness today:

One screwup:

One intention for tomorrow:

Why:

☐ Make others happy
☐ Show love & support
☐ Challenge myself
☐ Feel good/have fun
☐ Complete overdue task
☐ Resolve something
☐ Make progress
☐ Relax

"Thought is the sculptor who can create the person you want to be." **—HENRY DAVID THOREAU**

DATE: ___/___/___

One success I had today:

One redo I want:

One goal for tomorrow:

Why:

- ☐ Make others happy
- ☐ Show love & support
- ☐ Challenge myself
- ☐ Feel good/have fun
- ☐ Complete overdue task
- ☐ Resolve something
- ☐ Make progress
- ☐ Relax

"How do you know you're going to do something, until you do it?" —**J. D. SALINGER**

One happiness today:

One screwup:

One intention for tomorrow:

Why:

- ☐ Make others happy
- ☐ Show love & support
- ☐ Challenge myself
- ☐ Feel good/have fun
- ☐ Complete overdue task
- ☐ Resolve something
- ☐ Make progress
- ☐ Relax

DATE: __/__/__

"I consider that a man's brain originally is like a little empty attic, and you have to stock it with such furniture as you choose."
—ARTHUR CONAN DOYLE

Success of the week:

Best experience of the week:

One treat planned for the weekend:

One inspiration/realization:

MONDAY

DATE: __/__/__

"The dog that trots about finds a bone."
—GOLDA MEIR

One success I had today:

One redo I want:

One goal for tomorrow:

Why:

- ☐ Make others happy
- ☐ Show love & support
- ☐ Challenge myself
- ☐ Feel good/have fun
- ☐ Complete overdue task
- ☐ Resolve something
- ☐ Make progress
- ☐ Relax

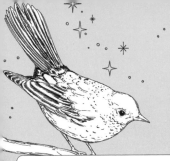

TUESDAY

DATE: __/__/__

"Self is a sea boundless and measureless."
—KAHLIL GIBRAN

One happiness today:

One screwup:

One intention for tomorrow:

Why:

- ☐ Make others happy
- ☐ Show love & support
- ☐ Challenge myself
- ☐ Feel good/have fun
- ☐ Complete overdue task
- ☐ Resolve something
- ☐ Make progress
- ☐ Relax

WEDNESDAY

DATE: __/__/__

"Poverty was the greatest motivating factor in my life." **—JIMMY DEAN**

One success I had today:

One redo I want:

One goal for tomorrow:

Why:

- ☐ Make others happy
- ☐ Show love & support
- ☐ Challenge myself
- ☐ Feel good/have fun
- ☐ Complete overdue task
- ☐ Resolve something
- ☐ Make progress
- ☐ Relax

DATE: __/__/__

"My friends are my 'estate.' Forgive me then the avarice to hoard them." **—EMILY DICKINSON**

One happiness today:

One screwup:

One intention for tomorrow:

Why:

- ☐ Make others happy
- ☐ Show love & support
- ☐ Challenge myself
- ☐ Feel good/have fun
- ☐ Complete overdue task
- ☐ Resolve something
- ☐ Make progress
- ☐ Relax

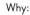

"I've always tried to go a step past wherever people expected me to end up." —**BEVERLY SILLS**

DATE: __/__/__

One success I had today:

One redo I want:

One goal for tomorrow:

Why:

- ☐ Make others happy
- ☐ Show love & support
- ☐ Challenge myself
- ☐ Feel good/have fun
- ☐ Complete overdue task
- ☐ Resolve something
- ☐ Make progress
- ☐ Relax

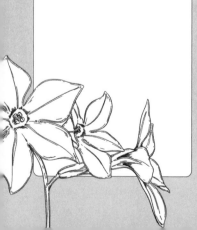

DATE: __/__/__

"We cannot all do everything." —**VIRGIL**

Success of the week:

Best experience of the week:

One treat planned for the weekend:

One inspiration/realization:

MONDAY

DATE: __/__/__

"Be thine own palace, or the world's thy jail."
—JOHN DONNE

One happiness today:

One screwup:

One intention for tomorrow:

Why:

- ☐ Make others happy
- ☐ Show love & support
- ☐ Challenge myself
- ☐ Feel good/have fun
- ☐ Complete overdue task
- ☐ Resolve something
- ☐ Make progress
- ☐ Relax

TUESDAY

DATE: ___/___/___

"Artistic growth is, more than it is anything else, a refining of the sense of truthfulness."
—WILLA CATHER

One success I had today:

One redo I want:

One goal for tomorrow:

Why:

- ☐ Make others happy
- ☐ Show love & support
- ☐ Challenge myself
- ☐ Feel good/have fun
- ☐ Complete overdue task
- ☐ Resolve something
- ☐ Make progress
- ☐ Relax

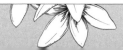

WEDNESDAY

DATE: __/__/__

"Do whatever you do intensely."
—ROBERT HENRI

One happiness today:

One screwup:

One intention for tomorrow:

Why:

- ☐ Make others happy
- ☐ Show love & support
- ☐ Challenge myself
- ☐ Feel good/have fun
- ☐ Complete overdue task
- ☐ Resolve something
- ☐ Make progress
- ☐ Relax

THURSDAY

"Better to light a candle than to curse the darkness."
—WILLIAM L. WATKINSON

DATE: __/__/__

One success I had today:

One redo I want:

One goal for tomorrow:

Why:

☐ Make others happy
☐ Show love & support
☐ Challenge myself
☐ Feel good/have fun
☐ Complete overdue task
☐ Resolve something
☐ Make progress
☐ Relax

"Crave for a thing, you will get it. Renounce the craving, the object will follow you by itself."
—SIVANANDA SARASWATI

DATE: __/__/__

One happiness today:

One screwup:

One intention for tomorrow:

Why:

- ☐ Make others happy
- ☐ Show love & support
- ☐ Challenge myself
- ☐ Feel good/have fun
- ☐ Complete overdue task
- ☐ Resolve something
- ☐ Make progress
- ☐ Relax

"*I am a big believer that you have to nourish any relationship.*" —**NANCY REAGAN**

DATE: __/__/__

Success of the week:

Best experience of the week:

One treat planned for the weekend:

One inspiration/realization:

"I come to win." —**LEO DUROCHER**

One success I had today:

One redo I want:

One goal for tomorrow:

Why:

- ☐ Make others happy
- ☐ Show love & support
- ☐ Challenge myself
- ☐ Feel good/have fun
- ☐ Complete overdue task
- ☐ Resolve something
- ☐ Make progress
- ☐ Relax

DATE: ___/___/___

"Grace has been defined as the the outward
expression of the inward harmony of the soul."
—WILLIAM HAZLITT

One happiness today:

One screwup:

One intention for tomorrow:

Why:

- ☐ Make others happy
- ☐ Show love & support
- ☐ Challenge myself
- ☐ Feel good/have fun
- ☐ Complete overdue task
- ☐ Resolve something
- ☐ Make progress
- ☐ Relax

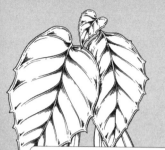

WEDNESDAY

DATE: __/__/__

"You have to learn the rules of the game. And then you have to play better than anyone else."
—UNKNOWN

One success I had today:

One redo I want:

One goal for tomorrow:

Why:

☐ Make others happy
☐ Show love & support
☐ Challenge myself
☐ Feel good/have fun
☐ Complete overdue task
☐ Resolve something
☐ Make progress
☐ Relax

DATE: __/__/__

"A pessimist is correct oftener than an optimist, but an optimist has more fun, and neither can stop the march of events." —**ROBERT A. HEINLEIN**

One happiness today:

One screwup:

One intention for tomorrow:

Why:

- ☐ Make others happy
- ☐ Show love & support
- ☐ Challenge myself
- ☐ Feel good/have fun
- ☐ Complete overdue task
- ☐ Resolve something
- ☐ Make progress
- ☐ Relax

DATE: __/__/__

"The weeds keep multiplying in our garden, which is our mind ruled by fear. Rip them out and call them by name." —**SYLVIA BROWNE**

One success I had today:

One redo I want:

One goal for tomorrow:

Why:

- ☐ Make others happy
- ☐ Show love & support
- ☐ Challenge myself
- ☐ Feel good/have fun
- ☐ Complete overdue task
- ☐ Resolve something
- ☐ Make progress
- ☐ Relax

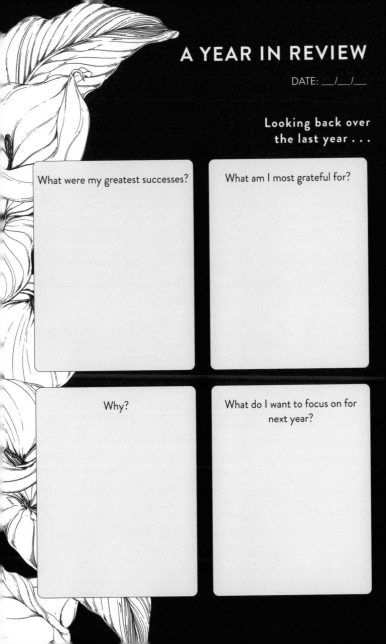

A YEAR IN REVIEW

DATE: __/__/__

**Looking back over
the last year . . .**

What were my greatest successes?

What am I most grateful for?

Why?

What do I want to focus on for
next year?

CONTRIBUTORS

Abloh, Virgil—Am. fashion designer

Adams, Joey—Am. comedian

Alcott, Louisa May—19th-cen. Am. novelist

Ali, Muhammad—Am. prizefighter

Andrews, Julie—Eng. actress

Angelou, Maya—Am. author & poet

Aragon, Louis—French poet

Aristotle—Ancient Greek philosopher

Ashe, Arthur—Am. tennis player

Asimov, Isaac—Am. author

Atlas, Charles—Ital.-Am. bodybuilder

Augustine, Norman Ralph—Am. businessman

Aurelius, Marcus—Roman emperor

Austen, Jane—Early 19th-cen. Eng. novelist

Bacall, Lauren—Am. actress

Ball, Lucille—Am. actress

Barrie, J. M.—Scot. novelist

Basie, Count—Am. jazz pianist

Basil of Caesarea—4th-cen. Byzantine bishop

Beall, Jerry S.—Am. writer

Beckett, Samuel—Irish playwright

Beecher Stowe, Harriet—19th-cen. Am. author

Beecher, Henry Ward—19th-cen. Am. minister & abolitionist

Bellow, Saul—Can.-Am. writer

Berle, Milton—Am. comedian

Berra, Yogi—Am. baseball player

Billings, Josh—19th-cen. Am. humorist

Blake, William—Late 18th-early 19th-cen. Eng. poet & artist

Bombeck, Erma—Am. humorist

Brazile, Donna—Am. political strategist

Brontë, Charlotte—19th-cen. Eng. novelist

Brooks, Phillips—19th-cen. Am. Episcopal clergyman & author

Brown, Brené—Am. professor & author

Brown, Les—Am. author

Browne, Sylvia—Am. author & psychic

Buddha, Gautama—founder of Buddhism

Burnett, Carol—Am. entertainer

Burroughs, James—Am. author

Burroughs, John—19th-cen. Am. naturalist

Buscaglia, Leo—Am. author

Caine, Mark—Am. analyst

Campbell, Joseph—Am. author

Camus, Albert—French philosopher

Carnegie, Dale—Am. business writer

Carver, George Washington—Am. scientist

Cather, Willa—Am. novelist

Cayce, Edgar—19th-cen. Am. clairvoyant

Cervantes, Miguel de—16th-cen. Span. writer

Chandler, Kyle—Am. actor

Churchill, Winston—Brit. prime minister

Clinton, Hillary—US secretary of state

Confucius—Ancient Chinese philosopher

Connolly, Billy—Eng. actor

Corddry, Rob—Am. actor

Cox, Marcelene—Am. writer

Dean, Jimmy—Am. country singer

Dewey, John—19th-cen. Am. philosopher

Dickinson, Emily—19th-cen. Am. poet

Diderot, Denis—18th-cen. French philosopher

Diller, Phyllis—Am. comedian

Diogenes, Laërtius—Ancient Greek biographer

Disney, Walt—Am. entrepreneur

Disraeli, Benjamin—19th-cen. Brit. prime minister

Donne, John—17th-cen. Eng. poet

Doyle, Arthur Conan—Eng. author

Drummond, Henry—19th-cen. Scottish evangelist

Dumas, Alexandre—19th-cen. French writer

Durocher, Leo—Am. baseball player & manager

Dyer, Wayne—Am. author

Earhart, Amelia—Am. aviator

Easwaran, Eknath—Indian spiritual author

Eckhart, Meister—Late 13th-cen. German theologian

Edison, Thomas A.—Am. inventor

Einstein, Albert—Ger.-Am. physicist

Eisenhower, Dwight D.—34th US president

Eliot, George—19th-cen. Eng. novelist

Elliot, Jim—Am. missionary

Elliot, Walter—Scot. politician

Emeagwali, Philip—Nigerian computer scientist

Emerson, Ralph Waldo—19th-cen. Am. essayist & philosopher

Epictetus—Ancient Greek philosopher

Feather, William—Am. author

Feltham, Owen—17th-cen. Eng. writer

Fey, Tina—Am. actress

Fisher, Carrie—Am. actress

Ford, Henry—19th-cen. Am. industrialist

France, Anatole—French poet

Francis of Assisi—13th-cen. Ital. friar & saint

Franklin, Benjamin—18th-cent. Am. polymath and statesman

Freud, Sigmund—Austrian psychoanalyst

Fuller, Buckminster—Am. architect & inventor

Fuller, Thomas—17th-cen. Eng. scholar, preacher & author

Gardner, John W.—US secretary of health

Garland, Judy—Am. actress

Gawain, Shakti—Am. author

Gervais, Ricky—Eng. comedian

Gibran, Khalil—Leb.-Am. writer & poet

Ginsberg, Allen—Am. poet

Goethe, Johann Wolfgang von—19th-cen. Ger. poet

Gracián, Baltasar—17th-cen. Span. writer

Gyatso, Tenzin—The 14th Dalai Lama

Hale, Edward Everett—19th-cen. Am. author

Hamilton, Laurell K.—Am. author

Harari, Yuval Noah—Israeli historian & author

Hazlitt, William—late 18th-cen. Eng. essayist

Hedberg, Mitch—Am. comedian

Heinlein, Robert A.—Am. science fiction author

Henri, Robert—Am. painter

Herbert, George—17th-cen. Eng. poet

Hill, Napoleon—Am. self-help author

Hinckley, Gordon B.—Am. LDS Church leader

Hitchcock, Alfred—Eng. filmmaker

Hodgson, Joel—Am. writer

Hood, Thomas—19th-cen. Eng. poet

Horace—Roman poet

Hubbard, Elbert—Am. writer

Hunt, H.L.—American political activist

Huxley, Aldous—Eng. writer & philosopher

Iglesias, Julio—Span. singer-songwriter

Iqbal, Muhammad—Pakistani poet

Jackson, Bo—Am. football & baseball player

James, William—19th-cen. Am. philosopher

Jefferson, Thomas—3rd US president

Jerome, Jerome K.—19th-cen. Eng. writer

Joan of Arc—15th-cen. Fr. saint

Johnson, Samuel—18th-cen. Eng. writer & lexicographer

Jones, Franklin P.—Am. humorist

Jowett, Benjamin—19th-cen. Eng. scholar & teacher

Jung, Carl—Swiss psychologist

Kalam, A. P. J. Abdul—Indian president

Kazantzakis, Nikos—Greek novelist

Keller, Helen—Am. author & disability rights advocate

Kennedy, John F.—35th US president

Kennedy, Rose—Am. philanthropist

Kiam, Victor—Am. entrepreneur

Kierkegaard, Søren—19th-cen. Danish philosopher

King, Elle—Am. singer-songwriter

Knight, Bobby—Am. basketball coach

Koontz, Dean—Am. author

La Bruyère, Jean de—17th-cen. French philosopherr

Lao Tzu—Ancient Chinese philosopher

Levenson, Sam—Am. humorist

London, Jack—Am. novelist

Lucas, George—Am. film director

Mandela, Nelson—S. Afr. president

Mandino, Og—Am. author

Marden, Orison Swett—19th-cen. Am. author

Marquis, Don—Am. humorist

Marshall, Peter—US Senate chaplain

Meir, Golda—Israeli prime minister

Montapert, Alfred A.—Am. author

Morley, Christopher—Am. journalist

Murray, Bill—Am. actor

Musk, Elon—S. Afr. entrepreneur

Nancherla, Aparna—Am. comedian

Nash, Ogden—Am. poet

Nathan, George Jean—Am. drama critic & editor

Nhat Hanh, Thich—Viet. Buddhist monk

Nightingale, Florence—19th-cen. nursing pioneer

Nin, Anaïs—Fr.-Am.-Cuban diarist

O'Connor, Flannery—Am. author

Paz, Octavio—Mex. poet

Peale, Norman Vincent—Am. minister

Persius—Roman poet

Pope, Alexander—18th-cen. Eng. poet

Posner, Michael I.—Am. psychologist

Rand, Ayn—Russ.-Am. writer

Reagan, Nancy—former US First Lady

Reeve, Christopher—Am. actor

Rilke, Rainer Maria—Austrian poet

Robbins, Tony—Am. author & motivational speaker

Rockefeller, John D.—Am. business magnate

Rogers, Will—Am. performer, humorist & cowboy

Rohn, Jim—Am. entrepreneur

Roosevelt, Eleanor—former US First Lady

Roosevelt, Theodore—26th US president

Rorty, Richard—Am. philosopher

Rowland, Helen—Am. journalist

Russell, Bertrand—Brit. philosopher & logician
Ruth, Babe—Am. baseball player
Salinger, J. D.—Am. author
Sandburg, Carl—Am. poet
Savitch, Jessica—Am. news anchor
Schuller, Robert H.—Am. televangelist
Schulz, Charles M.—Am. cartoonist
Schweitzer, Albert—Fr. theologian
Seinfeld, Jerry—Am. stand-up comedian and actor
Shakespeare, William—Late 16th-cen. Eng. poet & playwright
Sidney, Philip—16th-cen. Eng. poet
Sills, Beverly—Am. operatic soprano
Sivananda Saraswati—Indian yoga guru
Sophocles—Ancient Greek tragedian
Spinoza, Baruch—17th-cen. Dutch philosopher
Steinem, Gloria—Am. feminist & journalist
Stevenson, Robert Louis—19th-century Scot. novelist
Stone, Clement W.—Am. businessman

Stoppard, Tom—Czech-Brit. playwright
Swett Marden, Orison—19th-cen. Am. author
Swindoll, Charles R.—Am. evangelical pastor & author
Szasz, Thomas—Hung.-Am. psychiatrist
Tagore, Rabindranath—Indian poet
Teresa of Ávila—16th-cen. Span. nun & saint
Thoreau, Henry David—19th-cen. Am. transcendentalist
Tolle, Eckhart—German author & spiritual teacher
Twain, Mark—Late 19th-cen. Am. writer
Tyson, Cicely—Am. actress
van Dyke, Henry—Late 19th-cen. Am. author
Venturi, Ken—Am. golfer
Vidal, Gore—Am. writer
von Clausewitz, Carl—Early 19th-cen. Prussian general
vos Savant, Marilyn—Am. columnist
Washington, George—1st US president
Watkinson, William L.—Eng. author
Webster, Daniel—19th-cen. lawyer & US secretary of state

Weil, Simone—Fr. philosopher
Wells, H. G.—Eng. writer
Wharton, Edith—19th-cen. Am. novelist
White, Ron—Am. stand-up comedian
Whitefield, George—18th-cen. evangelist
Whitman, Walt—19th-cen. Am. poet
Wilde, Oscar—19th-cen. Irish poet & playwright
Wilson, Daniel—Am. singer-songwriter
Wilson, Flip—Am. comedian
Wilson, Harold—Brit. prime minister
Wilson, Woodrow—28th US president
Wodehouse, P. G.—Eng. author
Woolf, Virginia—Eng. author
Wordsworth, William—18th-cen. Eng. poet
Wright, Steven—Am. stand-up comedian
Yeats, John Butler—Irish artist
Yousafzai, Malala—Pakistani activist
Yutang, Lin—Chinese novelist, translator & philosopher
Zigler, Zig—Am. salesman & author
Zola, Émile—Fr. novelist
Zsa Zsa Gabor—Am. actress

ABOUT THE AUTHOR